Menopause

A Mental Health Practitioner's Guide

Menopause

A Mental Health Practitioner's Guide

Edited by

Donna E. Stewart, M.D., F.R.C.P.C.

Professor and Chair of Women's Health
University Health Network
University of Toronto
Toronto, Ontario, Canada

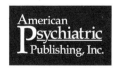

Washington, DC
London, England

Copyright © 2005 American Psychiatric Publishing, Inc.

ALL RIGHTS RESERVED

Manufactured in the United States of America on acid-free paper

09 08 07 06 05   5 4 3 2 1

First Edition

Typeset in Adobe's Berkeley, Formata, and Isadora Regular

American Psychiatric Publishing, Inc.
1000 Wilson Boulevard
Arlington, VA 22209–3901
www.appi.org

Library of Congress Cataloging-in-Publication Data
Menopause: a mental health practitioner's guide /edited by Donna E. Stewart.--1st ed.
    p. ; cm.
    Includes bibliographical references and index.
    ISBN 1-58562-160-9 (pbk. : alk. paper)
    1. Menopause. 2. Menopause--Psychological aspects. 3. Middle aged women--Mental health. 4. Middle aged women--Psychology.
    [DNLM: 1. Menopause--psychology. 2. Menopause--physiology. 3. Women--psychology. WP 580 M5466 2005] I. Stewart, Donna E., 1943– II. Title.
    RG186.M448 2005
    618.1'75--dc22

                                                            2004023832

British Library Cataloguing in Publication Data
A CIP record is available from the British Library.

Contents

Contributors

David A. Baram, M.D.
HealthPartners Medical Group, St. Paul, Minnesota; Assistant Clinical Professor of Obstetrics and Gynecology, University of Minnesota School of Medicine, Minneapolis, Minnesota

Angela M. Cheung, M.D., Ph.D., F.R.C.P.C.
Assistant Professor, Department of Medicine, and Associate Director, Women's Health, University Health Network, University of Toronto, Toronto, Ontario, Canada

Diana L. Dell, M.D., F.A.C.O.G.
Assistant Professor of Psychiatry and Behavioral Science and of Obstetrics and Gynecology, Duke University Medical Center, Durham, North Carolina

Khursheed Khine, M.D.
Clinical Fellow, Behavioral Endocrinology Branch, National Institute of Mental Health, Bethesda, Maryland

Jayashri Kulkarni, M.B.B.S., M.P.M., Ph.D., F.R.A.N.Z.C.P.
Professor of Psychiatry, Department of Psychological Medicine, Monash University, Alfred Hospital, Melbourne, Australia

Jamie A. Luff, M.D.
Clinical Fellow, Behavioral Endocrinology Branch, National Institute of Mental Health, Bethesda, Maryland

Jennifer Prouty, M.S.N., R.N.C.
Staff, Massachusetts General Hospital Center for Women's Mental Health, Boston, Massachusetts

Marta B. Rondon, M.D.
Assistant Professor, Department of Psychiatry and Mental Health, Universidad Peruana Cayetano Heredia and Hospital Nacional Edgardo Rebagliati M, EsSalud, Lima, Peru

David R. Rubinow, M.D.
Clinical Director and Chief, Behavioral Endocrinology Branch, National Institute of Mental Health, Bethesda, Maryland

Peter J. Schmidt, M.D.
Chief, Unit on Reproductive Endocrine Studies, Behavioral Endocrinology Branch, National Institute of Mental Health, Bethesda, Maryland

Claudio N. Soares, M.D., Ph.D.
Assistant Professor of Psychiatry, Harvard Medical School; Associate Director for Research, Massachusetts General Hospital Center for Women's Mental Health, Boston, Massachusetts

Meir Steiner, M.D., Ph.D., F.R.C.P.C.
Professor of Psychiatry and Behavioural Neurosciences and of Obstetrics and Gynecology, McMaster University, Hamilton, Ontario, Canada; Director of Research, Department of Psychiatry; and Director, Women's Health Concerns Clinic, St. Joseph's Healthcare, Hamilton, Ontario, Canada

Donna E. Stewart, M.D., F.R.C.P.C.
Professor and Chair of Women's Health, University Health Network, University of Toronto, Toronto, Ontario, Canada

Nada L. Stotland, M.D., M.P.H.
Professor of Psychiatry and Obstetrics/Gynecology, Rush Medical College, Chicago, Illinois

Preface

To every thing there is a season, and a time to every
   purpose under the heaven:
A time to be born and a time to die; a time to plant,
And a time to pluck up that which is planted;
A time to kill, and a time to heal; a time to break down,
   and a time to build up;
A time to weep, and a time to laugh; a time to mourn,
   and a time to dance.

Ecclesiastes 3:1–4 (New Revised Standard Version)

$\mathcal{M}$enopause is about change: change in reproductive status, hormone secretion, bodily function, appearance, expectations, relationships, and social circumstances. But it is also a normal life stage. Most women traverse the menopausal transition with little or no difficulty. Many welcome the cessation of menstruation and an end to risk of unwanted pregnancies, looking forward to new opportunities with an enthusiasm described by Margaret Mead as "postmenopausal zest."

There is, however, an inherent danger of pathologizing a normal life event in writing this book for mental health practitioners. The notion that women become irritable and depressed at menopause has long prevailed among both clinicians and women. Population data show that the menopausal years are not associated with an increased risk of depression for most women, and numerous studies have shown that psychosocial factors account more for the variation in the depressed mood of menopausal women than does menopause itself (Avis et al. 2001). The widely held view that the menopausal transition is usually associated with depression does a disservice to women because it raises negative expectations in women, their partners, employers, and physicians. For those women who do become depressed during this time of life, it leads them to consider depression to be a normal part of menopause and not seek appropriate treatment. However, increasing evidence suggests that in contrast to women in general, women seeking treatment for menopausal symptoms and a subset of women, especially those with previous depression, do appear to be particularly vulnerable to depression during the menopausal transition (Freeman et al. 2004; Stewart and Boydell 1993).

The changes associated with menopause are not limited to those that occur in women themselves. Ideas about the menopause are in flux. Indeed, even the definitions used to describe the different time periods and stages associated with natural (nonsurgical) menopause have changed over time and are still sometimes used in confusing ways. In this book, we will use the 1994 World Health Organization Scientific Group on Research in the Menopause terminology, augmented by the more recent refinements made by the Stages of Reproductive Aging Workshop (STRAW), which reminds us that "reproductive aging is a process, not an event, and that not all healthy women follow the same patterns. While most women will progress from one stage to the next, some women will see-saw back and forth between stages or skip a stage altogether" (Soules et al. 2001, p. 403). Not all women have symptoms as they transition to menopause, and women with symptoms experience them in different combinations and levels of intensity (Soules et al. 2001).

The anchor for most staging systems for reproductive senescence is the final menstrual period (FMP). The term *perimenopause* includes the time immediately prior to menopause (when the endocrinological, biological, and clinical factors of approaching menopause commence) and the first year after the FMP. Hence, *menopause* is a diagnosis that can only be made retrospectively (after 12 months of amenorrhea following the FMP). The term *menopausal transition* refers to the 1 or 2 years immediately prior to the FMP when the variability of the menstrual cycle is usually increased. In addition, STRAW further refined this classification by dividing the transition into *early* and *late* menopausal transition stages. The term *postmenopause* is defined as the time after the FMP, regardless of whether the menopause was induced or spontaneous (Utian 2001). STRAW also divided postmenopause into *early* (within 5 years of the FMP) and *late* stages (see Chapter 2, Physiology and Symptoms of Menopause, for details of menopausal staging and symptoms).

Enormous shifts in scientific knowledge and medical recommendations surrounding the management of perimenopause and menopause have occurred in the last decade. Hormone replacement therapy was advocated during the latter half of the 1990s as an essential aspect of well-woman care, for the prevention of heart disease, osteoporosis, and dementia, and as a general tonic. The publication in June 2002 of the Women's Health Initiative radically changed scientific and clinical opinion about the role of exogenous female hormones in menopause (Writing Group for the Women's Health Initiative Investigators 2002). New studies and analyses appear on a regular basis, leaving women and their physicians in a quandary about the best course to follow (Shumaker et al. 2004). Mental health practitioners also struggle to monitor new evidence as it emerges and to make optimal clinical decisions based on it. In this book, we describe the knowledge and clinical recommendations associated with menopause in 2004. The reader will need to continue to monitor new developments that may affect best practices in this area.

I have tried to organize this book in a way that would be most useful for mental health clinicians. The first chapter sets the contexts of midlife in women, and the second describes the basic physiology of the menopausal transition and menopause. Chapter 3 focuses on the effects of gonadal hormones on the central nervous system, setting the stage for Chapter 4, on depression, anxiety, and irritability during the menopausal transition and midlife. Attention has recently been paid to the effect of gonadal hormones and menopause on psychotic illness in women, and new research findings and clinical advice pertaining to this topic are in Chapter 5.

Mental health is intricately related to physical health: Chapter 6 looks at the medical aspects of perimenopause and menopause, and Chapter 7 at the gynecologic aspects of this time of life. Finally, Chapter 8 looks beyond menopause to the psychopathology and psychotherapy of older women in various cultures.

The authors have been selected from a pool of international menopause experts in psychiatry, neuroscience, gynecology, and internal medicine, and they cover the field from broad and diverse perspectives. I hope the timely information contained in this volume will be helpful to mental health professionals in formulating current best understanding and treatment for the psychological problems that a small percentage of women experience while traversing this life stage. If this is accomplished, then the goal of this book will have been met.

Donna E. Stewart, M.D., F.R.C.P.C.
Professor and Chair of Women's Health
University Health Network
University of Toronto
Toronto, Ontario, Canada

References

Avis NE, Stellato R, Crawford S, et al: Is there a menopausal syndrome? Menopausal status and symptoms across racial/ethnic groups. Soc Sci Med 52:345–356, 2001

Freeman EW, Sammel MD, Liu L, et al: Hormones and menopausal status as predictors of depression in women in transition to menopause. Arch Gen Psychiatry 61:62–70, 2004

Shumaker SA, Legault C, Kuller L, et al (WHIMS investigators): Conjugated equine estrogens and incidence of probable dementia and mild cognitive impairment in postmenopausal women: Women's Health Initiative Memory Study. JAMA 291:2947–2958, 2004

Soules MR, Sherman S, Parrott E, et al: Executive summary: Stages of Reproductive Aging Workshop (STRAW). Menopause 8:402–407, 2001

Stewart DE, Boydell KM: Psychologic distress during menopause: associations across the reproductive life cycle. Int J Psychiatry Med 23:157–162, 1993

Utian WH: Semantics, menopause-related terminology, and the STRAW reproductive aging staging system. Menopause 8:398–401, 2001

World Health Organization: Research on Menopause: Report of a WHO Scientific Group. WHO Technical Report Series 866. Geneva, World Health Organization, 1994

Writing Group for the Women's Health Initiative Investigators: Risks and benefits of estrogen plus progestin in healthy postmenopausal women: principal results from the Women's Health Initiative randomized controlled trial. JAMA 288:321–333, 2002

Chapter 1

The Contexts of Midlife in Women

Nada L. Stotland, M.D., M.P.H.

*M*idlife starts with a handicap; it is a euphemism. Menopause does not occur in the middle of life. Menopause means aging; aging is frightening; and so we pretend we are just halfway through life, rather than appreciating the maturity conferred by our years. This linguistic evasion reflects the dynamics and the context within which menopause occurs in the West. While women in some other cultures pay no particular attention to menopause, or experience it as an opportunity for greater freedom (Stewart 2003; Webster 2002), those in the Western world are preoccupied with it (Obermeyer 2000). Centuries of our history, folklore, and fairy tales have cast postmenopausal women as witches, hags, and crones. This is a book about menopause, and this "midlife" chapter focuses on the context of the perimenopausal period, approximately ages 40–55 years. Despite its technical inaccuracy, the term *midlife* will be used at some points in the chapter for convenience.

The recent scientific literature on menopause is overwhelmingly focused on hormonal changes, hormone administration, and their effects on general and gynecological health as well as mental health. However, there is a considerable body of knowledge about other facets of menopause that is useful for the mental health professional as well. Most mental health patients are women, and many adult women are either menopausal or contemplating menopause. In this book, we address the somatic changes that characterize the transition to menopause, the expanding knowledge base about the interactions between gonadal hormones and the central nervous system, general medical and gynecological aspects of this stage of life, the vicissitudes of behavioral or psychiatric symptoms and diseases during menopause, and psychopathology and psychotherapy for women moving beyond menopause into older age. These are crucial underpinnings for mental health treatment.

In addition to the challenges of linguistic, cultural, and age confusions, the perimenopausal period also encompasses a significant range of life stages. Some women are having their first babies when they are over age 40. Others are dealing with infertility. Some have made a considered decision not to have children. Some would have liked to have children in the context of a committed relationship but did not find a satisfactory relationship, or must make their peace with a lifelong inability to conceive. Despite sensationalized examples, for most women menopause is the end of fertility. There are also women who by 40 have teenagers or are grandmothers. Some women are focused on retirement; others are just beginning first, second, or third careers, or entering the workplace for the first time because of economic hardship or because they no longer have children at home. Last, the contexts of women's lives are diverse. In a chapter such as this, there is always the risk of focusing on mainstream American culture as though it were the only one, when, in fact, so-called minorities constitute a large proportion of the population in America, and other countries have their own traditions and circumstances.

A woman's experience of menopause is largely shaped by the psychological, social, and cultural context in which she lives; her observations; her expectations; and the expectations and reactions of important people in her life (Avis et al. 1997; Lock 1998; Olofsson and Collins 2000; Winterich and Umberson 1999). It was striking for this writer, as a Westerner, to visit a country in Asia and see people rush to help her (a perfectly strong and healthy Caucasian white-haired woman) onto a bus, or hear a man undergoing an appendectomy under acupuncture anesthesia report that he is honored that she is present, or have a waiter insist that she have the head of the duck—a great honor—at the end of a banquet. Observations such as these put Western attitudes and practices into relief and give us the opportunity to see them more clearly. Psychological, social, and cultural factors are closely interrelated (Kaufert 1996).

The Psychosocial Context

The overarching feature of the social context for midlife women is change. The roles of perimenopausal women in Western society have changed drastically over recent decades. The changes have occurred in the workplace, in leisure activities, in interpersonal relationships, and in the family.

The adaptation of women to new social mores can give rise to discomfiture in men unsure about the rules for their behavior. Just as women are caught between appearing weak but feminine and capable but masculine, men are caught between seeming distant and rude and being accused of patronizing or committing sexual harassment. Do they open doors for women? Pat women on the back when they do a good job? Compliment a woman on her appearance? Any circumstances that make one gender uncomfortable reverberate to the other gender. These issues are especially poignant for the generation of men and women during whose adulthood these issues came to the fore and who are now at midlife. Women still in, or thrust back into, the dating mode must make choices not available during their youth; this can be liberating or frightening.

The changing lives of midlife women reverberate throughout the family. Advising the next generation about pregnancy, childbirth, and parenting is an important and potentially gratifying role for a woman at midlife. However, there have been many changes in prenatal and birth care and customs. Many of today's grandmothers were advised to gain a minimal amount of weight but had few other prohibitions during their own pregnancies. They wore maternity clothes designed to camouflage their pregnancies. Their daughters are allowed to gain more weight but are strictly advised against eating raw seafood or rare meat, smoking, and drinking alcohol. They wear maternity tops designed to show off their bellies—or they leave their bellies uncovered. Today's American grandmothers may have had general anesthesia during labor or opted for natural childbirth. They stayed in the hospital for up to a week after birth. Their sons were circumcised. In contrast, their daughters are more likely to have epidurals, leave the hospital within a day after birth, and question the need for male circumcision. Grandmothers of little boys may never have seen an uncircumcised baby boy. Most Western women now at midlife did not breast-feed their babies; their daughters do. Naked pregnant bellies, uncircumcised penises, and breast-feeding are powerful psychological images and symbols that can provoke feelings ranging from envy to revulsion. These feelings, occurring just when women's daughters most need their support, can present a significant psychological challenge.

By midlife, most women are adept at running a household. Society, including many women, does not acknowledge women's domestic organizational duties. Credit is not given for mental tasks—only for physical tasks. Therefore, if a woman uses hired household help, household appliances, or prepared foods, it is assumed that her tasks have become significantly reduced. This is not so true in the working sphere, particularly for men. Secretaries and executive assistants are not presumed to relieve their bosses of their basic work duties. Supervising staff is considered a legitimate element of work. Running a household and caring for family is a major organizational job. At midlife, women are generally responsible for the feeding, clothing, and medical care of everyone in the family. They have to make major and minor decisions about family matters: where the children go to school, what extracurricular activities they engage in, whether they have made good relationships with suitable friends, whether social events will be organized, what they will be, who will be invited, and who will perform the necessary tasks. Some women just entering perimenopause had expected domestic tasks to be shared equally with male partners. Although there is more sharing than in the past, most of these women have learned that equal sharing is not to be. At the same time, in most countries, women still tend to be paid less for the same work (Misra 2001). They are more likely to be poor (Misra 2001).

There has been some recognition that midlife women are in a "sandwich generation," simultaneously responsible for adolescent children and aging adult relatives. Women are much more likely to care for family members, including their spouses, than are men. Many women have male partners significantly older than they are. As time goes by, many of these men become ill with heart disease, diabetes, malignancies, dementias, and other conditions. They are cared for by women, but women cannot anticipate the same level of care as they age. Approximately 10% of women are currently caring for a sick or disabled family member. Of these, half of those with incomes below $35,000 per year (in 1998) provide more than 20 hours of care per week, and only 18% have any paid home health care (Misra 2001). The incidence of depression among these women is high. Mental health professionals can help them recognize and satisfy their own needs for rest, relief, and care.

Today's grandmothers are much more likely to have spent years as full-time mothers than are their daughters. Between 1950 and 1998, the percentage of women in the labor force of the United States more than doubled, from 30% to more than 60% (Misra 2001). Statistics in other countries parallel these. Some women have to stifle their concerns about the effects of day care centers and employed mothers on their grandchildren. Some may resent the fact that the fathers of their daughters' children do not assume a fair share of domestic obligations; others may be uncomfortable when their sons or sons-in-law do housework or care for children.

The Workplace Context

The entry of most women into the paid workforce is a double-edged sword. It affects women in this age group in a variety of ways. Basic to many of them is the fact that the increase in women's occupational obligations has not been met with a commensurate diminution of their domestic obligations. Women are still responsible for the lion's share of domestic organization and tasks. Changing mores and opportunities have greatly diminished the availability of paid household help. The impact of household appliances, for those who have them, has been much smaller than is generally assumed. Whatever has been gained in the way of diminished labor intensity has been counterbalanced by increased task frequency. The rugs are not taken outside, hung on a line, and beaten in the spring and fall; they are vacuumed once or more often every week. The clothes and linens are not used for a week and then washed in a tub over a fire and hung on a line; they are changed every day or more often, as family members wear work or school clothes, athletic or exercise clothes, other casual garments, and sleepwear. There are loads and loads of laundry to do. There may be very little walking but a great deal of nerve-racking driving.

The range of experiences in the workplace for women at midlife is enormous. Some enjoy the opportunity to go back to school, change careers, or fulfill work plans they have had for years. Those who have been invested in their work for decades can find themselves ignored or replaced by younger employees. Others are hitting their stride, perhaps some years later than male colleagues. Some are coming to grips with the "glass ceiling" or other realities, and they are trying to accept limitations they had hoped to surpass. Still others are tired of working, or they may be satisfied with their employment achievements; either way, they are looking forward to retirement and opportunities to relax and enjoy family and new or postponed interests. Western European women may enjoy retirement benefits at earlier ages than women in other places. Economic difficulties in much of the world are forcing some women to continue employment for more years than they had intended.

The perimenopausal years can be very demanding for professional women. If they have not found a life partner, they must either decide to live an independent life or find a partner quickly from a very small pool of candidates. Women who have had children earlier in life may now be making up for lost time professionally just as their children become teenagers. Work challenges may be at their peak. A woman whose career accomplishments or earnings outstrip those of her male partner is expected to tread lightly to preserve his self-esteem. Some successful men are expected to have professionally accomplished wives, and some place a high premium on youth and attractiveness. In either case, they require an able hostess who is free to accompany them in work-related travel and entertainment activities. Women who handle all the demands gracefully, or appear to, inspire envy. Should the struggle become apparent, however, a woman may be seen as greedy and be accused of trying to "have it all." No such assertion is made about men who have both professions and children.

Women who were denied educational and occupational opportunities in their youth may feel demeaned by a society in which people are identified and judged by their occupations, as is common in North America (Calasanti and Slevin 2001) and less common in other parts of the world. These feelings may be exacerbated by the denigration of motherhood attributed, however inaccurately, to the feminist movement in North America. The intense mental and physical effort of childbearing and childrearing do not convey commensurate social status. Women are looked at askance if they choose not to have children and are blamed for their own infertility if they delay attempts at pregnancy until their educations are complete and their occupations and incomes established. Women may be encouraged to put off childbearing and then find themselves pushed aside in the workplace when they reach midlife. Midlife women may be in these situations themselves, or they may have daughters in these situations.

The Medical Context

The chapters of this book reflect the medicalization of the perimenopause in Western society. The advent of exogenous hormone treatments has exacerbated our society's tendency to consider menopause a disease rather than a normal physiological stage of life. Menopause has been regularly referred to in the medical literature as a deficiency state and a condition to be actively medically managed (Coney and Seaman 1994). Not long ago, women were bombarded with articles and radio and television presentations informing them that menopause is associated with a rise in cardiovascular disease, osteoporosis, and other conditions, and that hormone treatment can restore the health benefits associated with the premenopausal years. Penetration of these messages varied by ethnicity and socioeconomic status (Appling et al. 2000), as have the use of complementary and alternative approaches to menopause and new generations of medications (Bair et al. 2002; Fitzpatrick 1999).

Our preoccupation with the dire medical consequences of menopause, and the expectation that so-called replacement hormones will obviate those consequences, has even distorted our interpretation of actuarial data. Because women's average life expectancy a hundred years ago was approximately the same as the age of menopause, it has been argued, women were not meant by nature to survive beyond menopause. Life beyond menopause is an anomaly created by modern medicine. The fact is that average women's life expectancy a hundred years ago was drastically reduced by childhood diseases, other infectious diseases, and complications of pregnancy and childbirth (Misra 2001). Women who survived to menopause did not drop off and die. The survival of women beyond menopause is important to the survival of the species. If women could bear children until they died, they would not survive to mother the children born in the last several years of their lives, and they would not be available to mentor and care for coming generations. Children with grandmothers fare significantly better than those without them (Agee 2000).

Reports that the first large, prospective, controlled, and randomly assigned study of hormone therapy had yielded unanticipated negative outcomes threw some menopausal women and clinicians into consternation (Wenger et al. 2002; Writing Group for the Women's Health Initiative Investigators 2002). Because the study involved one particular hormone combination, there is controversy about the possibility that another formulation or regimen would offer benefits that outweigh the risks. Women abruptly withdrawn from hormones can suffer bouts of menopausal symptoms or symptoms they attribute to menopause, such as mood changes. The concept of menopause as a deficiency state has permeated their thinking, and women are now left with no way to remedy the perceived deficiency or forestall serious threats to their health. The promise of eternal, or at least prolonged, youth has been frustrated. Physicians are faced with the possibility of having harmed their patients by recommending and prescribing hormones, and with difficult questions about why they did so. Patients are faced with the negative images of aging that were fostered by the promotion of hormones— and with grave concerns about the trustworthiness of the medical establishment and their own doctors (Grodstein et al. 2003).

Some women, some health care professionals, some societies, and some countries (such as Japan) have been skeptical about hormonal medications from the beginning. Those who have substituted so-called natural hormone treatments, such as soy preparations, are at a loss; they have no way of knowing whether the cautions now associated with prescribed hormone preparations apply to them as well. Others feel that their refusal to accept the deficiency disease concept has been vindicated.

The Cultural Context

The meaning of menopause and the nature of the so-called generation gap vary from subculture to subculture and family to family within the larger society. The timing, nature, severity, and presumed importance of menopausal symptoms vary as well (Avis et al. 2001). The experience of menopausal symptoms is closely related to a woman's expectations of symptoms (Avis et al. 1997; Glazer et al. 2002; Koster et al. 2002; Mishra et al. 2002). Some cultures honor traditions in which women gain respect and support as they age. In others, women are marginalized as they age. Although few midlife women need help carrying out activities of daily living, the prospect of dependency casts a shadow over women who anticipate that they will have to move to nursing homes, with lonely and incompetent residents and callous staff, when they get older. Where cultural continuity is valued, there is little generation gap. Where "old-fashioned" ideas are denigrated in favor of "modern" lifestyles, older women can be perceived as irrelevant, if not burdensome.

Immigrants to North America, western Europe, and elsewhere come from many different countries and under many different circumstances. Some are refugees from war and inhuman treatment who have lost loved ones or seen them tortured. Others have left their countries of origin to seek better economic and educational opportunities for themselves and their children. Transcultural moves pose particular problems for midlife women. It is not as easy for them to learn new languages as it is for younger people. They are busy at home and at work, without the structure of school to foster their language skills and acculturation. Although young people may not have attained significant social status in their cultures of origin, and elderly people can be legitimately retired, midlife women often lose their careers in transit. They often have both children and elderly relatives to care for.

Native-born women live in many cultures as well. National leaders simultaneously laud the advent of opportunities for women and their representation in positions of leadership, and blame employed mothers for all the problems of their children and children in general. Women from cultures of poverty may not regard the opportunity to do paid work as an advance for themselves and their daughters. Generations of women in the family may have had to work at menial jobs to support their families. On the one hand, they may find themselves out of step with the work rhetoric of mainstream culture as they aspire for their daughters to have the luxury of full-time domesticity. On the other hand, they may regret their lack of educational and occupational opportunity and be extremely eager for their daughters to go as far as possible in school and obtain the most prestigious and well-paying jobs, whether their daughters wish to do so or not.

Given the worldwide economic downturn existing as this chapter is written, some women are disappointed that they cannot offer their children the financial and educational support they had hoped to. They may be unhappy that their adult children who have their own children need two incomes to survive and may be indefinitely impoverished or unable to buy their own homes. The disappointment is especially keen in societies like North American society, in which each generation is expected to reach a higher socioeconomic level than the one preceding. Women who had hoped to spend time with their grandchildren may have to go into, or stay in, the paid workforce. Women who had hoped to reenter or revitalize their working lives may find themselves with grandchildren to care for when their own children divorce, go back to school, or develop alcohol and substance abuse or legal problems.

The Context of Body Image

Most women in North America are dissatisfied with their bodies. This dissatisfaction begins to manifest itself shortly after toddlerhood. There are opposing forces affecting midlife women's body image. One is a preoccupation with decline and a dread of the loss of the youthful appearance that is synonymous with femininity in much of Western society. The other is a newfound sense of acceptance of one's body and liberation from the need to conform to social standards of appearance. The current emphasis on fitness can serve both forces: midlife women can use diet and exercise in an attempt to remain youthful and attractive, or they can experience midlife as a time when they allow themselves to try healthy new lifestyles and devote time and attention to their own bodies (Jamjan and Jerayingmongkol 2002). These are not mutually exclusive alternatives (Bloch 2002).

Exercise can be an excellent way to improve the body, body image, and general health while reducing stress. Of course, in some societies exercise for the sake of exercise is an alien concept, and in some of these, daily life requires a great deal of exercise.

Although women have an unprecedented life expectancy and can remain vigorous for decades after menopause, physical abilities do tend to decline with age. Many women need to use reading glasses for the first time. Arthritis affects one joint or another. Breasts sag. Wrinkles appear. Changes in appearance, at any time of life, require adjustment and adaptation (Ransdell et al. 1998). Losses of function naturally cause some dismay; in our society, however, they frequently also lead to ridicule. Hot flashes advertise a woman's personal perimenopausal status to intimate partners, family members, and work colleagues.

Where age brings respect, signs of aging may be welcome. In the Western world, increasing numbers of women seek botulinum toxin or collagen injections, plastic surgery, and other means to forestall the appearance of aging. Some Western women choose to accept signs of aging gracefully; others would like to postpone them a bit; and some become desperate to hide them.

These issues are fertile ground for psychotherapeutic exploration.

Overweight is another cause for derision in Western society. The prevalence of obesity in midlife women is large and growing, cutting across all sectors of society but especially affecting women who are poor and/or members of minority groups (Laferrere et al. 2002; Shaw et al. 2000). There is a major clash between social expectations and reality. We know that the increased incidence of obesity is related to changes in our diet, and we know that overweight is associated not only with poor body image but also with poor health, but there is little evidence that any medical treatment, aside from surgical diminution of the gastrointestinal tract, successfully produces lasting weight reduction. Clinicians as well as patients are in a quandary. Overweight patients may look to clinicians to encourage and facilitate weight loss, but those who fail to lose weight may be reluctant to see their clinicians for other care important to their overall health. Recently, there has been a movement for self-acceptance among overweight women.

The Sexual Context

Attitudes toward the sexuality of midlife women have clustered at two poles. On one side, women are expected to lose their sexuality as they lose their fertility. They are considered neither sexually interested nor sexually attractive. On the other side, women are vibrantly sexual through midlife and until death. As with all polarized attitudes, these are grossly oversimplified and unhelpful (Daniluk 1995).

The refusal to recognize or accept sexuality throughout the life span has deprived us of accurate information about women's feelings and behaviors (Kingsberg 2002). It may make women reluctant to engage in sexual activity and potential partners reluctant to approach them. It deters midlife women from seeking medical advice for sexual problems and causes their health care professionals to be both embarrassed and uninformed. The media emphasis on ongoing sexual interest, along with freedom from concerns about conception and the heightened self-confidence that can come with maturity, has enabled some women to enjoy sex more in their midlife years than they did when they were younger. They can be more self-assertive and eager to try new techniques (Hallstrom and Samuelsson 1990).

Making sexuality in midlife legitimate opens more possibilities for women, but not if it raises unrealistic expectations in them and in society (Dennerstein et al. 1999). Media depictions accompanying stories about, or hinting at, women's midlife sexuality are very narrow. There are always a male and female partner of approximately the same age. They are trim, fit, active, and happy. Unfortunately, many women are not trim, fit, or happy;

many lack male partners; and some are interested in homosexual, rather than heterosexual, intimacy. Thinning and dryness of the vaginal lining as a result of decreasing estrogen levels complicate intercourse (Barlow et al. 1997). Studies of midlife women's sexuality have focused on sexual intercourse and orgasm rather than including the whole range of sexual interest and expression (Laumann et al. 1999; Modelka and Cummings 2003). As men age, some turn to younger women, leaving same-aged partners behind. Women tend to live longer than men, but the availability of younger male partners is limited by social disapproval and the attitudes of younger men themselves.

Divorce, remarriage, and stepchildren are prominent features of contemporary life frequently involving women at midlife. For example, approximately half of the marriages in North America end in divorce, most within the first few years of marriage, but many later on as well. Most women know of a relationship that began with two young people struggling to make their way, with the wife supporting the man financially as well as emotionally, then taking responsibility for the children and household while he advanced professionally and financially, only to be left for a younger woman after 20 or 30 years. To seek new emotional and sexual partners, midlife women must bridge the gap between the dating and sexual mores of their youth and those predominant now.

In the wealthy Western world, the advent of medications for male erectile dysfunction brought some sexual issues for women to the fore. We learned that male impotence had deprived many interested women of the opportunity for sexual intercourse with their male partners. We also learned that their male partners' impotence had been a relief to other women, who had viewed sexual relations with their partners as a burdensome but otherwise inescapable obligation. Recent interest in testosterone or other treatments may inspire some women to look for ways to maintain and enhance decreasing libido and sexual gratification, but it may also make women who had been perfectly satisfied with some decrease in sexual activity feel inadequate (Padero et al. 2002). The clinician working with midlife women must take special care to avoid assumptions and biases while instead providing accurate information as it becomes available and fostering a therapeutic atmosphere in which the whole range of sexual concerns, activities, interests, and abilities can be entertained and addressed (Rice 2001).

Clinical Applications: The Mental Health Context

The material in this chapter is a strong rationale for a basic clinical rule: Make no assumptions. Women at midlife are an enormously diverse group:

in sexual orientation, ethnicity, intimate relationships, childbearing and parenting, sexual interest and behavior, employment, socioeconomic status, and general health. A patient in a lesbian relationship may have been married and had children, and she may have concurrent or intermittent heterosexual relationships. A well-educated, well-off patient may be a current victim of domestic violence. A patient who is a member of a sexually abstinent religious order may have had an active sexual life in the past. A patient may be pleased to be entering the most satisfying phase of her sexual life or pleased that her sexual obligations are over. Many patients will have concerns about exogenous hormones and what the shifting recommendations imply in terms of the reliability of other medical advice. The mental health clinician can supply scientific information and support patients' informed personal preferences.

The relationship between menopause and depression is still a debated issue, to be discussed in Chapter 4, Mood Disorders, Midlife, and Reproductive Aging. Suffice it to say here that menopause is probably, in and of itself, not a precipitant of depression in most women (Bebbington et al. 2003). Despite all the stressors noted above, midlife women enjoy comparatively good health. Although some regret the departure of their children into independent lives, most are relieved to have fulfilled those parental obligations and, after menopause, to have put the possibility of pregnancy and the need for contraception behind them. They feel more sure of themselves and less concerned about the opinions of others than they did earlier in their lives (Busch et al. 2003; Dennerstein et al. 2002). Menopause can be a time for self-reflection. Awareness that life is finite can make life richer. Plans long postponed can be implemented: further education, new careers, travel, hobbies. Perimenopausal women are a gratifying population to work with. The clinician can draw on and enhance patients' mature capacities, resulting from years of life experience, along with the flexibility of a life stage called "the change" and the likelihood of many remaining years in which to enjoy the fruits of treatment.

References

Agee E: Menopause and the transmission of women's knowledge: African American and white women's perspectives. Med Anthropol Q 14:73–95, 2000

Appling SE, Allen JK, Van Zandt S, et al: Knowledge of menopause and hormone replacement therapy use in low-income urban women. J Womens Health Gend Based Med 9:57–64, 2000

Avis NE, Crawford SL, McKinlay SM: Psychosocial, behavioral, and health factors related to menopause symptomatology. Women Health 3:103–120, 1997

Avis NE, Stellato R, Crawford S, et al: Is there a menopausal syndrome? Menopausal status and symptoms across racial/ethnic groups. Soc Sci Med 52:345–356, 2001

Bair YA, Gold EB, Greendale GA, et al: Ethnic differences in use of complementary and alternative medicine at midlife: longitudinal results from SWAN participants. Am J Public Health 92:1832–1840, 2002

Barlow DH, Cardozo LD, Francis RM, et al: Urogenital ageing and its effect on sexual health in older British women. Br J Obstet Gynaecol 104:87–91, 1997

Bebbington P, Dunn G, Jenkins R, et al: The influence of age and sex on the prevalence of depressive conditions: report from the National Survey of Psychiatric Morbidity. Int Rev Psychiatry 15:74–83, 2003

Bloch A: Self-awareness during the menopause. Maturitas 41:61–68, 2002

Busch H, Barth-Olofsson AS, Rosenhagen S, et al: Menopausal transition and psychological development. Menopause 10:179–187, 2003

Calasanti T, Slevin K: Gender, Social Inequalities, and Aging. Walnut Creek, CA, AltaMira Press, 2001, pp 84–87

Coney S, Seaman B: The Menopause Industry: How the Medical Establishment Exploits Women. Alameda, CA, Hunter House, 1994

Daniluk J: Women's Sexuality Across the Life Span: Challenging Myths, Creating Meanings. New York, Guilford, 1995

Dennerstein L, Lehert P, Burger H, et al: Factors affecting sexual functioning of women in the mid-life years. Climacteric 2:254–262, 1999

Dennerstein L, Lehert P, Guthrie J: The effects of the menopausal transition and biopsychosocial factors on well-being. Arch Women Ment Health 5:15–22, 2002

Fitzpatrick LA: Selective estrogen receptor modulators and phytoestrogens: new therapies for the postmenopausal woman. Mayo Clin Proc 74:601–607, 1999

Glazer G, Zeller R, Delumba L, et al: The Ohio Midlife Women's Study. Health Care Women Int 23:612–630, 2002

Grodstein F, Clarkson TB, Manson JE: Understanding the divergent data on postmenopausal hormone therapy. N Engl J Med 348:645–650, 2003

Hallstrom T, Samuelsson S: Changes in women's sexual desire in middle life: the longitudinal study of women in Gothenburg. Arch Sex Behav 19:259–268, 1990

Jamjan L, Jerayingmongkol P: Self-image of people in their fifties. Nurs Health Sci 4 (3 suppl):A4, 2002

Kaufert PA: The social and cultural context of menopause. Maturitas 23:169–180, 1996

Kingsberg SA: The impact of aging on sexual function in women and their partners. Arch Sex Behav 31:431–437, 2002

Koster A, Eplov LF, Garde K: Anticipations and experiences of menopause in a Danish female general population cohort born in 1936. Arch Women Ment Health 5:9–13, 2002

Laferrere B, Zhu S, Clarkson JR, et al: Race, menopause, health-related quality of life, and psychological well-being in obese women. Obes Res 10:1270–1275, 2002

Laumann EO, Paik A, Rosen RC: Sexual dysfunction in the United States: prevalence and predictors. JAMA 281:537–544, 1999

Lock M: Menopause: lessons from anthropology. Psychosom Med 60:410–419, 1998

Mishra G, Lee C, Brown W, et al: Menopausal transitions, symptoms and country of birth: the Australian Longitudinal Study on Women's Health. Aust N Z J Public Health 26:563–570, 2002

Misra D: The Women's Health Data Book: A Profile of Women's Health in the United States, 3rd Edition. Washington, DC, Jacobs Institute, 2001

Modelka K, Cummings S: Female sexual dysfunction in postmenopausal women: systematic review of placebo-controlled trials. Am J Obstet Gynecol 188:286–293, 2003

Obermeyer CM: Menopause across cultures: a review of the evidence. Menopause 7:184–192, 2000

Olofsson ASB, Collins A: Psychosocial factors, attitude to menopause and symptoms in Swedish perimenopausal women. Climacteric 3:33–42, 2000

Padero MC, Bhasin S, Friedman TC: Androgen supplementation in older women: too much hype, not enough data. J Am Geriatr Soc 50:1131–1140, 2002

Ransdell LB, Wells CL, Manore MM, et al: Social physique anxiety in postmenopausal women. J Women Aging 10:19–39, 1998

Rice S: Sexuality and intimacy for aging women: a changing perspective, in Women as They Age, 2nd Edition. Edited by Garner JD, Mercer S. Binghamton, NY, Haworth, 2001, pp 147–164

Shaw JM, Ebbeck V, Snow CM: Body composition and physical self-concept in older women. J Women Aging 12:59–75, 2000

Stewart DE: Menopause in highland Guatemalan women. Maturitas 44:293–297, 2003

Webster RW: Aboriginal women and menopause. J Obstet Gynaecol Can 24:938–940, 2002

Wenger NK, Paoletti R, Lenfant CJM, et al (eds): International position paper on women's health and menopause: a comprehensive approach (NIH Publ No 02–3284). Bethesda, MD, National Institutes of Health, 2002

Winterich JA, Umberson D: How women experience menopause: the importance of social context. J Women Aging 11:57–73, 1999

Writing Group for the Women's Health Initiative Investigators: Risks and benefits of estrogen plus progestin in healthy postmenopausal women: principal results from the Women's Health Initiative randomized controlled trial. JAMA 288:321–333, 2002

Chapter 2

Physiology and Symptoms of Menopause

David A. Baram, M.D.

$\mathcal{I}$n this chapter, I review the following topics: 1) the age at onset of menopause and factors that may affect this, 2) the endocrinology of the menopausal transition, and 3) the symptoms of the menopausal transition. In the last decade, two large studies have greatly expanded our knowledge of the epidemiologic and symptomatic aspects of the menopausal transition.

Age at Onset of Perimenopause and Menopause

The best data available on the age at onset of perimenopause and menopause come from the Massachusetts Women's Health Study (MWHS), a 5-year prospective, longitudinal, population-based study of 2,570 women (McKinlay 1996; McKinlay et al. 1992), and the Study of Women's Health Across the Nation (SWAN), based on 16,063 multiethnic women in a cross-sectional study and 3,306 women in the longitudinal study now in its tenth year (Avis et al. 2001; Santoro 2004). In addition to answers to questions about the age at onset of the perimenopause and menopause and the signs and symptoms of menopause, the MWHS recorded women's attitudes as they went through the menopausal transition. (See the preface to this volume for a definition of terms based on menopausal staging.) The MWHS found that the majority of women in the survey had positive feelings about menopause; 42% of the women in the study reported feeling relieved when menstruation ceased, and 35.5% reported neutral feelings. Some women (19.6%) reported mixed feelings about menopause, but only 2.7% of the women in the sample expressed regret when menstruation ceased. Negative feelings about menopause were more common in women who were depressed, had severe menopausal symptoms such as hot flashes and insomnia, or had previous negative attitudes and expectations about menopause.

Perimenopause is the phase in the aging process when women pass from reproductive to nonreproductive life (Burger et al. 2002; Jones and Muasher 1994; Speroff 2002). Perimenopause includes the period immediately prior to menopause (when the endocrinological, biological and clinical features of approaching menopause commence) and the first year after the final menstrual period (FMP). At this stage of life, the ovaries become relatively resistant to the stimulatory effects of the pituitary gonadotropins follicle-stimulating hormone (FSH) and luteinizing hormone (LH). During the perimenopause, women often have menstrual irregularity, longer and heavier menstrual periods, and prolonged episodes of amenorrhea. In addition to changes in the menstrual cycle, the perimenopause is marked by decreased (but not absent) fertility, vasomotor symptoms (hot flashes), psychological changes, insomnia, and changes in sexual function (Bachmann 1994; Santoro 2002).

The Stages of Reproductive Aging Workshop (STRAW) divided perimenopause into "early" and "late" menopausal transition stages. The early menopausal transition stage is characterized by regular menstrual cycles, but the length changes by 7 days or more (e.g., every 21 days instead of 28 days). The late menopausal transition stage is characterized by two or more skipped menstrual cycles and at least one intermenstrual interval of 60 days or more. Both early and late menopausal transition stages are accompanied by elevated FSH levels and variable levels of symptoms (Soules et al. 2001).

Data from the MWHS indicate that the perimenopausal transition usually begins about 4 years before the FMP (McKinlay 1996; McKinlay et al. 1992; Speroff 1994) and that the median age at onset of perimenopause is 47.5 years. In the MWHS, smokers were noted to have a shorter perimenopause than nonsmokers (McKinlay et al. 1992). Most women in the MWHS (90%) noted menstrual irregularity for years before their FMP; the other 10% had less than 6 months of menstrual irregularity before menopause or noted that their periods stopped abruptly and without warning (McKinlay 1996; Taffe and Dennerstein 2002). Change in the length of the menstrual cycle is primarily a result of an increase or decrease in the length of the follicular phase of the cycle. During the perimenopause, FSH levels are increased (>20 IU/L), inhibin B is decreased, LH levels are normal, and estradiol levels are slightly increased in response to elevated levels of FSH (Speroff 2002).

Menopause is the time in a woman's life when, after the depletion or atrophy of all gonadotropin-sensitive ovarian follicles, menstruation permanently ceases. Menopause is usually diagnosed retrospectively on a clinical basis, after the woman has experienced her FMP—that is, after 12 consecutive months of amenorrhea. Elevated FSH concentrations (>40 IU/L) are sometimes used to diagnose menopause, but studies have reported that postmenopausal concentrations of FSH sometimes can be found in regularly cycling perimenopausal women (Burger 1994). Therefore, menopause cannot be diagnosed solely on the basis of an elevated concentration of FSH (Barnes and Hajj 1993).

In the MWHS, the median age at onset of menopause was 51.3 years (range: 47–55 years). Although the median age at menarche has decreased significantly worldwide as a result of improved nutrition and better health care, the age at onset of menopause has remained the same since the time of ancient Greece (Speroff et al. 1999). The MWHS found that women who currently smoke experience menopause 1.5–2 years earlier than women who do not smoke. There is evidence of a dose–response relationship between the age at onset of menopause and the number of cigarettes smoked and duration of smoking. Former smokers and women who live at high altitudes also have an earlier onset of menopause (Midgette and Baron 1990; Speroff 1994). Cigarette smoking may cause an earlier onset of menopause by 1) exerting a direct toxic effect on ovarian follicles, 2) interfering with the hypothalamic-pituitary-ovarian axis, or 3) affecting the metabolism of the reproductive hormones (Midgette and Baron 1990; Whiteman et al. 2003). Lower educational attainment; nonemployment; a history of heart disease; and being separated, widowed, or divorced are associated with earlier natural menopause (Avis and McKinlay 1995; Speroff 2002). A lifetime history of depression may be associated with earlier menopause. Women with longstanding depression may experience dysfunction of the hypothalamic-pituitary-ovarian axis and an earlier decline of ovarian function compared with women who are not depressed (Harlow et al. 2003). Thinner or malnourished women and vegetarians experience an earlier menopause, probably because they have less body fat available for the conversion of androstenedione to estrogen. Women who consume alcohol have a later menopause as a result of higher levels of estrogen. Other factors associated with later age of natural menopause include parity, prior use of oral contraceptives, and Japanese ethnicity (Gold et al. 2001).

Menopause occurred before age 40 in about 1% of women in SWAN.

This condition is known as *premature ovarian failure* and is usually idiopathic. Higher body mass index and smoking are associated with premature menopause (Santoro 2004). Eating disorders, excessive exercise, and polycystic ovarian disorder can also cause premature menopause. Premature ovarian failure can be caused (rarely) by autoimmune disease (especially thyroid and adrenal disease) and is associated with myasthenia gravis, idiopathic thrombocytopenic purpura, rheumatoid arthritis, vitiligo, and autoimmune hemolytic anemia (Speroff et al. 1999). Women who experience natural menopause prior to age 40 have a 50% higher mortality rate than women who experience menopause at age 50 or older. This observed association between earlier age at menopause and mortality may be because of genetic factors, behavioral and environmental exposures, or other health-related factors (Gold et al. 2001).

Occasionally, younger women may experience oligomenorrhea, menopausal symptoms, and infertility because of a diminished number of ovarian follicles. When FSH concentrations are measured in these women, they may temporarily be in the menopausal range (>40 IU/L). Some of these women may begin to menstruate and ovulate again (after their FSH returns to the premenopausal range), and they may eventually become pregnant.

The term *postmenopause* is defined as dating after the FMP (Utian 2001). STRAW divides the postmenopause into "early" and "late" stages. Early postmenopause occurs in the 5 years after the FMP and encompasses a further dampening of the ovarian hormone function to a permanent level as well as a period of accelerated bone loss. The late stage begins 5 years after the FMP and ends with death (Soules et al. 2001).

Endocrinology of the Menopausal Transition

Perimenopausal Changes

Changes in the concentration and ratio of the reproductive hormones begin many years before menopause and are probably caused by several factors. The primary factor is a decrease in the number of functioning ovarian follicles as a result of ovarian atresia. The number of ovarian follicles decreases from an estimated high of 7 million during embryonic life to about 2 million at birth. Of the remaining follicles, about 400–500 are ovulated during the reproductive period of life, and the remainder are lost through atresia. Other factors that lead to changes in reproductive hormones during the perimenopause include resistance of the remaining ovarian follicles to gonadotropin stimulation (the "better" or more responsive ovarian follicles may be used earlier in life) and alterations in the sensitivity of the hypothalamic-pituitary-ovarian axis to changing estrogen concentrations (Longcope 1999; Metcalf et al. 1982; Santoro 2002; Speroff et al. 1999). Perimenopausal hormonal changes often commence when women are in their mid-30s and are partially responsible for the decreased fertility noted by women in their 30s and 40s (Hade and DeCherney 2000). In addition, as women age, their menstrual cycles increase in length, become more irregular (menstrual cycles are most regular during middle reproductive life), and are often anovulatory (Hee et al. 1993; Speroff 2002; Speroff et al. 1999).

The first detectable hormonal change of the perimenopause is a rising concentration of FSH and a declining concentration of inhibin B (Jones and Muasher 1994; Sherman et al. 1976), as shown in Figure 2–1. The rising FSH concentration is probably caused by a decrease in the number of gonadotropin-sensitive ovarian follicles, which stimulates the pituitary gland to produce more FSH in an effort to stimulate the resistant follicles. At the same time, the circulating concentrations of inhibin B (but not inhibin A) begin to decrease (Burger et al. 2002; Santoro 2002). Inhibin A is produced by the granulosa cells of the dominant follicle and the corpus luteum (Zapantis and Santoro 2003). Inhibin B, a sensitive measure of ovarian function, is produced by early, small antral follicles. Inhibin B and estrogen both have a negative feedback effect on FSH, and as the aging ovary produces less inhibin B and estradiol, the amount of FSH produced by the pituitary gland increases. The production of inhibin B begins to decrease at about age 35, reflecting a decreasing number of ovarian follicles, and stops completely at menopause (Burger et al. 2002; Hee et al. 1993).

During the early perimenopausal phase, while FSH is increasing and inhibin B is decreasing, the concentration of LH remains in the normal range. Late in the perimenopause, LH concentrations increase slightly but at a slower rate than those of FSH (LH has a much shorter half-life than FSH). The concentration of estrogen (primarily estradiol) remains in the normal range until approximately 1 year before menopause, when it gradually begins to decline (MacNaughton et al. 1992; Speroff 2002; Trevoux et al. 1986). Once menopause has occurred and all of the ovarian follicles have been depleted, estrogen concentrations decline precipitously.

Later in the perimenopause, FSH concentrations continue to rise, which has a significant effect on the menstrual cycle. The elevated FSH concentrations noted during the early follicular stage of each perimenopausal menstrual cycle cause unusually rapid follicular development and a relative decrease in the concentration of circulating follicular-phase estrogen. In addition, the follicular phase of the menstrual cycle becomes shorter. In the late perimenopausal phase, as transitory ovarian failure occurs, menstrual cycles become increasingly irregular, and many of the cycles become anovulatory (Taffe and Dennerstein 2002). At this time, luteal-phase defects

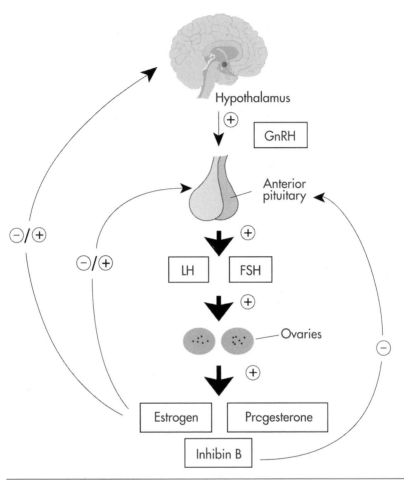

FIGURE 2–1.   Female hypothalamic-pituitary-ovarian axis

FSH=follicle-stimulating hormone; GnRH=gonadotropin-releasing hormone; LH= luteinizing hormone.

caused by decreased progesterone production by the corpus luteum are common, and conception becomes increasingly rare. Menstrual cycle length often increases to 35–42 days.

As noted earlier in this chapter, elevated—or postmenopausal—concentrations of FSH and LH and decreased concentrations of estradiol and progesterone can be detected before ovarian function ceases permanently (Hee et al. 1993). In other words, the hormonal profile of perimenopausal women during times of prolonged amenorrhea can be similar to the hormonal profile of postmenopausal women (Burger 1994; Hee et al. 1993). Therefore, perimenopausal women with elevated FSH concentrations can still become pregnant, and they should be cautioned to use birth control to avoid unplanned pregnancy until both LH and FSH concentrations are consistently and permanently elevated.

Postmenopausal Changes

With the onset of menopause, ovarian production of estrogen (both estradiol and estrone), progesterone, androstenedione, and testosterone decreases significantly. Estrogen concentrations decline significantly once menstruation ceases permanently, which leads to atrophy of estrogen-sensitive tissue (i.e., breast, bladder, skin, and internal and external genitalia). The loss of the negative feedback of estrogen on the pituitary gland leads to a dramatic increase in the production of FSH and LH as the gonadotropins attempt to stimulate the unresponsive ovarian follicles. In postmenopausal women, FSH production increases 10- to 20-fold, and LH production increases threefold. Gonadotropin concentrations reach maximum levels 1–3 years after menopause and then decrease slowly during the remaining postmenopausal years (Speroff 2002; Speroff et al. 1999).

After all of the ovarian follicles have been depleted, the ovary stops producing significant amounts of estrogen. However, the stroma of the postmenopausal ovary is stimulated by high levels of gonadotropins and continues to produce testosterone and smaller amounts of androstenedione (Longcope 1999). Most of the estrogen found in postmenopausal women is derived from the peripheral conversion of adrenal (70%) and ovarian (30%) androstenedione to estrone. Estradiol is the primary estrogen found in women during the reproductive years, whereas estrone is the primary estrogen noted in postmenopausal women. Some of the estrone produced by the peripheral conversion of androstenedione is converted to estradiol. The peripheral conversion of androstenedione to estrogens by aromatization takes place primarily in adipose tissue but also occurs in muscle, skin, and the liver. Therefore, overweight or obese women are hyperestrogenic when compared with thin women and are more likely to develop estrogen-dependent neoplasia, especially adenocarcinoma of the endometrium (Speroff et al. 1999). After menopause, there is no further corpus luteum formation, and the ovary no longer produces progesterone. The small amount of progesterone detectable in postmenopausal women is secreted exclusively by the adrenal gland (Metcalf et al. 1982).

In addition to the testosterone produced by the ovary, androgens are produced by the postmenopausal adrenal gland. The amount of dehydroepiandrosterone (DHEA) and its sulfate (DHEA-S) produced by the adrenal gland decreases after menopause. However, a report from SWAN shows an increase in DHEA-S from early to late menopausal transition of 9.6%, versus a decline from premenopause to early transition (Santoro 2004). After menopause, estrogen production declines more significantly than androgen production, and for this reason, the androgen-to-estrogen ratio changes significantly in postmenopausal women. The production of sex hormone–binding globulin also decreases after menopause, leaving more unbound circulating testosterone. This change in the androgen-to-estrogen ratio may be responsible for the facial hirsutism and loss of scalp hair noted by some postmenopausal women (Gass 1993; Speroff et al. 1999).

Toward the end of life, androstenedione production by the adrenal gland decreases significantly. In turn, little estrogen is produced by peripheral conversion of androgens, and estrogen-responsive tissue atrophies further.

Symptoms of Menopausal Transition

In addition to changes in the menstrual cycle, perimenopausal and menopausal women often report a number of general physical and emotional symptoms. These symptoms occur more frequently in women who experience hot flashes, especially if the flashes are severe. Physical symptoms include headaches, backaches, swelling, shortness of breath, breast sensitivity, weight gain, thinning of the skin, dizziness, palpitations, formication, and muscle and joint pain. Emotional symptoms include (in order of decreasing frequency) irritability, fatigue, tension, nervousness, depression, lack of motivation, insomnia (or early morning awakening), and feelings of isolation (Anderson et al. 1987; Dennerstein et al. 2000; Oldenhave and Netelenbos 1994; Oldenhave et al. 1993). It is often difficult to determine whether these symptoms are caused by hormonal or psychosocial factors.

Symptoms of the menopausal transition are decreased in women who are better educated, enjoy better self-rated physical and psychological health, do not experience premenstrual dysphoric disorder, use fewer over-the-counter medications, do not suffer from chronic medical conditions, have a lower level of interpersonal stress, do not smoke or consume excessive amounts of alcohol, exercise regularly, and have a positive attitude toward aging and the menopause (Dennerstein et al. 2000). Race also appears to play a role in the reporting of symptoms during menopause (Gold et al. 2004). Caucasian women report more psychosocial symptoms and African American women report more vasomotor symptoms.

Vulvovaginal Symptoms and Anatomical Changes

Common vulvovaginal symptoms found in postmenopausal women include irritation, itching, burning, and dyspareunia (difficult and painful intercourse) caused by vaginal atrophy. See Chapter 7, Gynecologic Aspects of Perimenopause and Menopause, for further information. A chronic vaginal discharge caused by a change in the vaginal environment from acidic to alkaline is common during menopause. Extensive vulvovaginal atrophy often causes bleeding, sometimes with only a light touch. A sensation of pressure in the vagina and pelvis may be caused by a cystocele (hernia of the bladder), a rectocele (hernia of the rectum), an enterocele (hernia of the intestine), or uterine prolapse. Aging results in loss of skin collagen and subcutaneous fat, which causes wrinkling of the skin and thinning of the labia majora and mons pubis. Loss and thinning of pubic hair are also common. Although most of the vulvovaginal symptoms noted above are caused by urogenital atrophy, more serious conditions always must be ruled out. The differential diagnosis of pelvic bleeding, pain, pressure, or burning should include benign and malignant neoplasms, vulvar dystrophies, infections, trauma, foreign bodies, and allergic reactions (Bachmann et al. 1999).

Both the vulva and the vagina contain a rich supply of estrogen receptors (Waggoner 1993). Therefore, vulvovaginal atrophy begins during the perimenopausal years as estrogen levels begin to wane. The vulva in peri- and postmenopausal women loses collagen and adipose tissue and becomes thinner, flattened, and less elastic (Bachmann 1994). The secretions of the vulvar sebaceous glands diminish, and the clitoris becomes smaller and less sensitive to touch. The prepuce of the clitoris atrophies, which causes clitoral irritation when the clitoris is stimulated during sexual arousal and intercourse. Many women notice that the dryness, irritation, burning, and itching caused by vulvar atrophy make them uncomfortable during the day and interfere with sleep at night.

The postmenopausal vagina loses rugae and becomes smooth and atrophic, and the vaginal walls appear smooth, friable, and pale. The alkaline vaginal environment and loss of glycogen from the vagina do not support the growth of the lactobacilli commonly found in the acidic premenopausal vagina; thus, postmenopausal women are more susceptible to vaginal infections (Bachmann et al. 1999; Gass 1993). Because the vascularity and the collagen content of the vagina decrease and the mucosa thins, the vagina becomes more friable and more susceptible to trauma and infection. The vagina loses length, diameter, and distensibility. These structural changes, along with the decrease in the amount of vaginal lubrication produced during sexual arousal, make dyspareunia a common problem in older women. Regular use of vaginal estrogen cream or estrogen-containing vaginal rings may reduce burning, itching, and dyspareunia. Use of lubricants before intercourse may also decrease dyspareunia.

Because of the friability of the vaginal mucosa, bleeding is common whenever the vaginal mucosa is traumatized, such as during speculum insertion or intercourse. As the postmenopausal vagina undergoes anatomical changes, the urethral meatus moves closer to the introitus, often resulting in dysuria. Increased urinary frequency, urinary urgency, and urinary tract infections may be associated with sexual intercourse.

As estrogen levels decline with the cessation of menses, the endometrium becomes atrophic, and the uterus and cervix decrease significantly in size. These anatomical changes occur gradually over time and continue throughout the lifetime of the woman. Uterine fibroids, which are dependent on estrogen stimulation for growth, often diminish dramatically in size when women stop menstruating. Therefore, women with symptomatic uterine fibroids may want to delay surgical treatment until the effect of menopause on the size of the fibroids can be assessed. The cervical os becomes stenotic, and the transformation zone of the cervix moves upward into the endocervical canal, making it more difficult to obtain sufficient cellular material for a Pap smear.

After menopause, the ovaries decrease significantly in size and are barely palpable during bimanual examination. Because postmenopausal women are anovulatory, functional cysts (corpus luteum cysts and follicular cysts) should not form in the ovaries. Therefore, any mass in the ovaries of postmenopausal women must be further evaluated to rule out the possibility of ovarian carcinoma.

The breasts of postmenopausal women lose support and subcutaneous fat, decrease in size, and lie flatter against the chest wall (Gass 1993). Breast parenchyma is eventually totally replaced with fatty tissue. The breast areola also decreases in size after menopause.

The estrogen deprivation that occurs at the onset of menopause can contribute to a decrease in the strength of the connective tissue and muscles supporting the uterus, bladder, and rectum (Hajj 1993). As women age, the ligaments supporting the pelvic viscera become more lax, allowing uterine prolapse (procidentia), cystocele, enterocele, and rectocele to develop. These anatomical changes, which are more common in multiparous women, may eventually cause pelvic pressure and discomfort, stress urinary incontinence, and difficulty emptying the bowel.

Stress and urge urinary incontinence can cause significant changes in a woman's lifestyle, leading to social withdrawal and isolation, avoidance of lovemaking, and curtailment of physical activity. When bathroom facilities are not readily available, women with urinary incontinence may have difficulty traveling, working, and shopping. Women with incontinence often must carefully plan trips away from home and must carry a change of clothing and locate bathrooms ahead of time. Common emotional responses to incontinence include depression, guilt, denial, anxiety, secretiveness, and fear that others will discover the patient's difficulty or smell her urine (Thiede 1992).

Hot Flashes

Hot flashes (or flushes) are the most reliable indicator of the perimenopause and menopause, the most frequently reported menopausal symptom (Swartzman et al. 1990), and one of the most distressing symptoms for perimenopausal and menopausal women (Barton et al. 2001; Freedman 2000; Kronenberg 1994). See also Chapter 7, Gynecologic Aspects of Perimenopause and Menopause. A hot flash is "a sudden, transient sensation ranging from warmth to intense heat that spreads over the body, particularly on the chest, face, and head, typically accompanied by flushing, perspiration, and often followed by a chill. In some instances, there are palpitations, and feelings of anxiety" (Kronenberg 1994, p. 97). In addition, some women experience vertigo and weakness during a hot flash (Ginsburg 1994). Many women experience an aura or prodromal sensation consisting of anxiety, tingling, or head pressure that precedes the hot flash by 5–60 seconds.

Significant risk factors for menopausal hot flashes include earlier age at onset of menopause, premenstrual dysphoric disorder, surgical menopause, African American ethnicity, and less than 12 years of education (Dennerstein et al. 2000; McKinlay et al. 1992; Schwingl et al. 1994; Stearns et al. 2002). Past or current alcohol consumption places women at higher risk of developing hot flashes. Contrary to previous studies that showed that increased fat protects women from vasomotor symptoms, data from SWAN show that a higher body mass index, smoking, decreased physical activity, and low socioeconomic status are significantly associated with more vasomotor symptoms (Santoro 2004). Parity and age at first and last pregnancy were not related to hot flashes at the time of menopause (Schwingl et al. 1994). In the MWHS, women who had fewer general physical symptoms before menopause and more positive attitudes toward menopause were less likely to report hot flashes (McKinlay et al. 1992).

What causes hot flashes? Although no exact etiology has been found, several investigators suggest that changes in the thermoregulatory set point located in the anterior portion of the hypothalamus are most likely responsible (Fitzpatrick and Santen 2002; Speroff 2002; Stearns et al. 2002). It has been demonstrated that women who experience hot flashes have a narrower thermoneutral zone (the core body temperature range within which sweating and shivering do not occur) compared with women who do not experience hot flashes (Freedman and Blacker 2002). Therefore, it takes only a small increase in core body temperature to precipitate a hot flash in symptomatic women. A hot flash begins with an increase in core body temperature. Women respond to the increase in core body temperature by attempting to cool down through sweating, cutaneous vasodilation (responsible for the flushing), and changes in behavior leading to a cooler environment. These physiological and behavioral cooling mechanisms then return core body temperature to normal, ending the hot flash (Freedman 2001; Shanafelt et al. 2002; Stearns et al. 2002).

The role of estrogen and other hormones and centrally acting neurotransmitters in the etiology of hot flashes is unknown. However, the association of estrogen deficiency and withdrawal with hot flashes can be inferred from the impressive effectiveness of estrogen therapy (ET) for hot flashes (Barton et al. 2001; Freedman and Blacker 2002). Estrogen therapy probably abates hot flashes by expanding the thermoneutral zone, thus raising the core body temperature sweating threshold (Freedman and Blacker 2002). Estrogen withdrawal decreases levels of endorphins and catecholamines, which leads to an increase in secretion of norepinephrine and serotonin from the hypothalamus. Norepinephrine and serotonin then lower the set point in the thermoregulatory nucleus in the hypothalamus, leading to a lowering of the core body temperature and the triggering of heat-loss mechanisms (Shanafelt et al. 2002).

Although most hot flashes are temporally associated with an increase in gonadotropin-releasing hormone (GnRH) and LH (but not FSH) levels, there does not seem to be a causal relationship between the pulsatile release of GnRH and LH and the onset of a hot flash. Indeed, hot flashes can occur in women who have undergone hypophysectomy (removal of the pituitary).

The sweating noted at the start of a hot flash usually is accompanied by an increase in finger temperature, a decrease in skin resistance, and an increase in skin conductance (Kronenberg 1994; Swartzman et al. 1990). At times, sweating can be profuse, causing clothing to become literally soaked. Heart rate, cutaneous blood flow, and skin temperature increase during the hot flash, but blood pressure does not change significantly. Cutaneous vasodilation, sweating, and attempts by the woman to cool off (e.g., taking off clothing, opening windows, moving to a cooler environment) cause heat loss and a slight lowering of core body temperature, often precipitating a chilling sensation, vasoconstriction, and actual shivering. Skin temperature then gradually returns to normal, often taking as long as 30 minutes (Kronenberg 1994).

A hot flash lasts from several seconds to a few minutes, with the average hot flash lasting 4 minutes (Fitzpatrick and Santen 2002; Speroff et al. 1999). The frequency of hot flashes and the way in which hot flashes are experienced also vary, both within and among individual women (Kronenberg 1994). Some women sweat profusely, whereas others do not. Symptoms in any woman may, of course, change over time. Hot flashes often occur spontaneously without any obvious precipitant; however, they can be triggered in some women by psychological stress, hot and humid weather, caffeine, alcohol, or certain foods (Kronenberg 1994).

Most American women experience hot flashes during the menopausal transition (Avis and McKinlay 1995; McKinlay et al. 1992; Schwingl et al. 1994). However, in the MWHS, 23% of the postmenopausal women never had hot flashes or night sweats. The prevalence of hot flashes can vary considerably depending on the population studied. Japanese women, who have been studied extensively, rarely report hot flashes, perhaps because of cultural expectations, genetic differences, or the plant estrogen they receive naturally from their diet (Lock et al. 1988).

Women often report hot flashes before they develop menstrual irregularity. The MWHS (Avis and McKinlay 1995; McKinlay et al. 1992) found that 10% of women had hot flashes before the final menstrual period. The peak time for reporting hot flashes, when they were experienced by 50% of the women in the study, occurred late in the perimenopause, just prior to the onset of the FMP. Women in the MWHS who did have hot flashes noted that the flashes were most prevalent during the first 2 years after menopause and that they decreased over time. Only 20% of the women in the MWHS were still experiencing hot flashes 4 years after their FMP. Women with a perimenopause of less than 6 months (about 10% of the MWHS sample) had a much lower prevalence of hot flashes—about 30%—than did women with a longer perimenopause.

The majority of women in the MWHS who experienced hot flashes (approximately 68%) reported that they were not bothered by them. Only 32% of the women in the study consulted a physician for treatment of menopausal symptoms, usually because their hot flashes or night sweats were frequent and severe and caused insomnia. However, hot flashes, especially those that are severe and persist for a long time, can be quite troublesome and embarrassing for some women. Women often need to modify their behavior or environment (e.g., by wearing light clothing or changing the room temperature) to accommodate the profuse sweating that accompanies hot flashes.

Women who have hot flashes are often awakened at night and are twice as likely to report insomnia as women who do not have hot flashes (Erlik et al. 1981). Women who have difficulty sleeping because of hot flashes often report irritability and fatigue the next day (Moe 1999; Shaver et al. 1988). Insomnia caused by hot flashes is the primary reason that women seek medical care and ET during the menopausal transition (Kronenberg 1994). Insomnia and daytime drowsiness affect productivity, safety at home and at work, and susceptibility to illness and depression (Moe 1999).

The beneficial effects of ET on sleep include reduction in insomnia, shorter time to get to sleep (sleep latency), and fewer episodes of wakefulness during the night. In addition, ET in women with hot flashes increases the amount of time spent in deeper and more restful rapid eye movement sleep (Erlik et al. 1981; Schiff et al. 1979). Estrogen therapy improves temperature regulation and restores disrupted circadian rhythms and melatonin production. It also decreases stress reactivity. With improved sleep patterns, women report less anxiety and improved ability to function socially (Schiff et al. 1979). See Chapter 6, Medical Aspects of Perimenopause and Menopause, and Chapter 7, Gynecologic Aspects of Perimenopause and Menopause, for more discussion of hormone therapy.

Sleep problems in aging women may not be entirely caused by changes in hormonal status, given that sleep difficulties often continue long after hot flashes have subsided (Moe 1999). Some sleep problems may be associated with sleep apnea, which is more common in overweight women and women with periodic limb movement disorders (Kravitz et al. 2003). Women tend to gain weight as they age, because of a decrease in energy expenditure and a decrease in resting metabolic rate (Santoro 2002).

Women who experience hot flashes prior to the menopausal transition should be evaluated for thyroid disease, pheochromocytoma, carcinoid, leukemia, and other carcinomas (Speroff et al. 1999).

Irregular Menstrual Bleeding

During the perimenopausal transition, changes in the typical menstrual cycle pattern often occur. See also Chapter 7, Gynecologic Aspects of Perimenopause and Menopause. Some women may develop anovulatory or dysfunctional uterine bleeding (DUB), which is characterized by irregular menstrual periods (metrorrhagia), intermenstrual spotting, excessive and prolonged menstrual periods (menorrhagia), and episodes of amenorrhea. A diagnosis of DUB implies that the bleeding comes from the endometrium and is not caused by a neoplastic process in the endometrial cavity or by a medical illness (Speroff et al. 1999). Shortened menstrual cycle intervals are caused by a decrease in the length of the follicular phase of the cycle (Gass 1993). Most of the perimenopausal changes in the menstrual cycle are caused by anovulation. If ovulation does not occur, no corpus luteum is formed, and no progesterone is available to bring about secretory changes to the endometrium. High sustained levels of estrogen, unopposed by the effects of progesterone, can cause an abnormal thickening of endometrial tissue that eventually leads to irregular ripening and shedding of the endometrium. After many years, unopposed estrogen stimulation of the endometrium can result in adenomatous hyperplasia or endometrial carcinoma (Speroff et al. 1999).

Endometrial hyperplasia or carcinoma should be suspected in all patients with postmenopausal bleeding (bleeding after 1 year of amenorrhea). These patients should be referred to a gynecologist to be evaluated with hysteroscopy and a full endometrial curettage to rule out neoplasms.

After any neoplastic process has been ruled out, perimenopausal anovulatory uterine bleeding can be managed with the administration of a short course of progesterone alone (either in oral or in intramuscular depot form). In low-risk perimenopausal women (those who do not smoke, do not have dyslipidemia, are not hypertensive, and do not have any other contraindication to the use of estrogen), continuous daily administration of a low-dose oral contraceptive can also be useful and is a good choice if contraception is desired. Women on that regimen who continue to bleed may be prescribed a trial of danazol (Danocrine) or the intramuscular depot form of a GnRH agonist by their gynecologist. However, GnRH agonists can only be used for a total of 6 months because they accelerate bone loss. Another useful gynecologic treatment is the placement of a progesterone-containing intrauterine device. These devices can be kept in place for 5 years, and they have been shown to decrease or eliminate menstrual bleeding in a significant number of women. If medical therapy fails to control DUB, endometrial ablation should be considered. Newer endometrial ablation techniques are extremely rapid and can often be used with local anesthesia and conscious sedation. Hysterectomy should be used only after all of the treatments listed here have failed.

Conclusion

The median age at onset of menopause is 51.3 years, with perimenopause beginning about 4 years earlier. Decreases in the number of functioning ovarian follicles, increased resistance of the remaining follicles to gonadotropin stimulation, and alterations in the sensitivity of the hypothalamic-pituitary-ovarian axis to changing estrogen concentrations all contribute to the changes in the concentrations and ratios of the reproductive hormones that herald the beginning of the menopausal transition. Symptoms reported include vasomotor instability (hot flashes), irregular menstrual bleeding, and urinary difficulties because of urogenital atrophy.

References

Anderson E, Hamburger S, Liu JH, et al: Characteristics of menopausal women seeking assistance. Am J Obstet Gynecol 156:428–433, 1987

Avis NE, McKinlay SM: The Massachusetts Women's Health Study: an epidemiologic investigation of the menopause. J Am Med Womens Assoc 50:45–49, 63, 1995

Avis NE, Stellato R, Crawford S, et al: Is there a menopausal syndrome? Menopausal status and symptoms across racial/ethnic groups. Soc Sci Med 52:345–356, 2001

Bachmann GA: The changes before "the change." Postgrad Med 95:113–124, 1994

Bachmann GA, Ebert GA, Burd ID: Vulvovaginal complaints, in Treatment of the Postmenopausal Woman: Basic and Clinical Aspects. Edited by Lobo RA. New York, Lippincott Williams & Wilkins, 1999, pp 195–202

Barnes R, Hajj SN: Pathophysiology of menopause, in Clinical Postreproductive Gynecology. Edited by Hajj SN, Evans WJ. Norwalk, CT, Appleton & Lange, 1993, pp 31–35

Barton D, Loprinzi C, Wahner-Roedler D: Hot flashes: aetiology and management. Drugs Aging 18:597–606, 2001

Burger HG: The menopause: when it is all over or is it? Aust N Z J Obstet Gynaecol 34:293–295, 1994

Burger HG, Dudley EC, Robertson DM, et al: Hormonal changes in the menopause transition. Recent Prog Horm Res 57:257–275, 2002

Dennerstein L, Dudley EC, Hopper JL, et al: A prospective population-based study of menopausal symptoms. Obstet Gynecol 96:351–358, 2000

Erlik Y, Tataryn IV, Meldrum DR, et al: Association of waking episodes with menopausal hot flushes. JAMA 245:1741–1744, 1981

Fitzpatrick LA, Santen RJ: Hot flashes: the old and the new, what is really new? Mayo Clin Proc 77:1155–1158, 2002

Freedman RR: Hot flashes revisited. Menopause 7:3–4, 2000

Freedman RR: Physiology of hot flashes. Am J Hum Biol 13:453–464, 2001

Freedman RR, Blacker CM: Estrogen raises the sweating threshold in postmenopausal women with hot flashes. Fertil Steril 77:487–490, 2002

Gass M: Physiology and pathophysiology of the postmenopausal years, in Gynaecology and Obstetrics: A Longitudinal Approach. Edited by Moore TR, Reiter RC, Rebar RW, et al. New York, Churchill Livingstone, 1993, pp 883–896

Ginsburg ES: Hot flashes—physiology, hormonal therapy, and alternative therapies. Obstet Gynecol Clin North Am 21:381–390, 1994

Gold EB, Bromberger J, Crawford S, et al: Factors associated with age at natural menopause in a multiethnic sample of midlife women. Am J Epidemiol 153:865–874, 2001

Gold EB, Block G, Crawford S, et al: Lifestyle and demographic factors in relation to vasomotor symptoms: baseline results from the Study of Women's Health Across the Nation. Am J Epidemiol 159:1189–1199, 2004

Hade JJ, DeCherney AA: Sex steroid hormone metabolism in the climacteric woman, in The Menopause: Comprehensive Management, 4th Edition. Edited by Eskin BA. New York, Parthenon, 2000, pp 87–96

Hajj SN: Pelvic relaxation and procidentia, in Clinical Reproductive Gynaecology. Edited by Hajj SN, Evans WJ. Norwalk, CT, Appleton & Lange, 1993, pp 112–117

Harlow BL, Wise LA, Otto MW, et al: Depression and its influence on reproductive endocrine and menstrual cycle markers associated with perimenopause. Arch Gen Psychiatry 60:29–36, 2003

Hee J, MacNaughton J, Bangah M, et al: Perimenopausal patterns of gonadotrophins, immunoreactive inhibin, oestradiol and progesterone. Maturitas 18:9–20, 1993

Jones GS, Muasher SJ: Hormonal changes in the perimenopause, in The Menopause: Comprehensive Management, 3rd Edition. Edited by Eskin BA. New York, McGraw-Hill, 1994, pp 257–268

Kravitz HM, Ganz PA, Bromberger J, et al: Sleep difficulty in women at midlife: a community survey of sleep and the menopausal transition. Menopause 10:19–28, 2003

Kronenberg F: Hot flashes, in Treatment of the Postmenopausal Woman: Basic and Clinical Aspects. Edited by Lobo RA. New York, Raven, 1994, pp 97–117

Lock M, Kaufert P, Gilbert P: Cultural construction of the menopausal syndrome: the Japanese case. Maturitas 10:317–332, 1988

Longcope C: The endocrinology of the menopause, in Treatment of the Postmenopausal Woman: Basic and Clinical Aspects. Edited by Lobo RA. New York, Lippincott Williams & Wilkins, 1999, pp 35–42

MacNaughton J, Banah M, McCloud P, et al: Age related changes in follicle stimulating hormone, luteinizing hormone, oestradiol and immunoreactive inhibin in women of reproductive age. Clin Endocrinol (Oxf) 36:339–345, 1992

McKinlay SM: The normal menopause transition: an overview. Maturitas 23:137–145, 1996

McKinlay SM, Brambilla DJ, Posner JG: The normal menopause transition. Maturitas 14:103–115, 1992

Metcalf MG, Donald RA, Livesey JH: Pituitary-ovarian function before, during and after the menopause: a longitudinal study. Clin Endocrinol (Oxf) 17:489–494, 1982

Midgette AS, Baron JA: Cigarette smoking and the risk of natural menopause. Epidemiology 1:475–480, 1990

Moe KE: Reproductive hormones, aging, and sleep. Semin Reprod Endocrinol 17:339–348, 1999

Oldenhave A, Netelenbos C: Pathogenesis of climacteric complaints: ready for the change? Lancet 343:649–653, 1994

Oldenhave A, Jaszmann LJ, Haspels AA, et al: Impact of climacteric on well-being. Am J Obstet Gynecol 168:772–780, 1993

Santoro N: Textbook of Perimenopausal Gynecology. Boca Raton, FL, CRC Press, 2002

Santoro N: What a SWAN can teach us about menopause. Contemp Ob Gyn 49:69–79, 2004

Schiff I, Regestein Q, Tulchinsky D, et al: Effects of estrogens on sleep and psychological state of hypogonadal women. JAMA 242:2405–2407, 1979

Schwingl PJ, Hulka BS, Harlow SD: Risk factors for menopausal hot flashes. Obstet Gynecol 84:29–34, 1994

Shanafelt TD, Barton DL, Adjei AA, et al: Pathophysiology and treatment of hot flashes. Mayo Clin Proc 77:1207–1218, 2002

Shaver J, Giblin E, Lentz M, et al: Sleep patterns and stability in perimenopausal women. Sleep 11:556–561, 1988

Sherman BM, West JH, Korenman SG: The menopausal transition: analysis of LH, FSH, estradiol, and progesterone concentrations during menstrual cycles of older women. J Clin Endocrinol Metab 42:629–636, 1976

Soules MR, Sherman S, Parrott E, et al: Executive summary: Stages of Reproductive Aging Workshop (STRAW). Menopause 8:402–407, 2001

Speroff L: The menopause: a signal for the future, in Treatment of the Postmeno- pausal Woman: Basic and Clinical Aspects. Edited by Lobo RA. New York, Raven, 1994, pp 1–8

Speroff L: The perimenopause. Definitions, demography, and physiology. Obstet Gy- necol Clin North Am 29:397–410, 2002

Speroff L, Glass RH, Kase NG: Clinical Gynecologic Endocrinology and Infertility, 5th Edition. Baltimore, MD, Williams & Wilkins, 1999

Stearns V, Ullmer L, Lopez JF, et al: Hot flushes. Lancet 360:1851–1861, 2002

Swartzman LC, Edelberg R, Kemmann E: The menopausal hot flush: symptom re- ports and concomitant physiological changes. J Behav Med 13:15–30, 1990

Taffe JR, Dennerstein L: Menstrual patterns leading to the final menstrual period. Menopause 9:32–40, 2002

Thiede HA: Psychosocial factors, in Female Pelvic Floor Disorders: Investigation and Management. Edited by Benson JT. New York, WW Norton, 1992, pp 179–184

Trevoux R, De Brux J, Castanier M, et al: Endometrium and plasma hormone profile in the peri-menopause and post-menopause. Maturitas 8:309–326, 1986

Utian WH: Semantics, menopause-related terminology, and the STRAW reproductive aging staging system. Menopause 8:398–401, 2001

Waggoner SE: Vulva and vagina, in Clinical Postreproductive Gynecology. Edited by Hajj SN, Evans WJ. Norwalk, CT, Appleton & Lange, 1993, pp 159–176

Whiteman MK, Staropoli CA, Langenberg PW, et al: Smoking, body mass, and hot flashes in midlife women. Obstet Gynecol 101:264–271, 2003

Zapantis G, Santoro N: The menopausal transition: characteristics and management. Best Pract Res Clin Endocrinol Metab 17:33–52, 2003

Chapter 3

Effects of Reproductive Hormones and Selective Estrogen Receptor Modulators on the Central Nervous System During Menopause

Claudio N. Soares, M.D., Ph.D.

Meir Steiner, M.D., Ph.D., F.R.C.P.C.

Jennifer Prouty, M.S.N., R.N.C.

Hormone Changes and Brain Functioning: Where Is the Bridge?

Several studies provide robust evidence that gonadal steroids can affect brain systems known to mediate depression and anxiety on multiple levels. The sexual dimorphism seen in hypothalamic-pituitary-adrenal axis regulation and the response to stress observed in animal studies and in humans corroborate this observation. The impact of sex hormones on brain functioning has been frequently cited as one of the factors that reinforce gender differences observed in the prevalence, outcome, and response to treatment of mental disorders. It is noteworthy that such differences become more noticeable with the onset of puberty and physical maturation, when young females undergoing physical and hormonal changes frequently report affective instability as well as higher levels of emotional distress. After puberty, gender proportions of depression and anxiety significantly change, with female-to-male ratio increasing to 2:1–3:1 (Born and Steiner 2001; Kessler et al. 1994; Steiner 1992). In addition, subgroups of women seem to be particularly vulnerable for developing depression during periods of heightened hormonal variability (i.e., premenstrual periods, puerperium, and perimenopause) (Harlow et al. 1999, 2003; Soares et al. 2001b; Stewart and Boydell 1993).

The occurrence of abrupt hormonal changes such as those observed during perimenopause, the subsequent onset of clinical symptoms, and the emergence of mood symptoms and cognitive deficits constitute a complex puzzle that awaits better explanation. In the 1990s, a community-based, prospective study, the Harvard Study of Moods and Cycles, was designed to explore some of the particularities regarding the association between depression and ovarian failure. In this study, more than 5,000 premenopausal women (ages 36–44) were initially invited to complete a self-administered screening questionnaire, in an attempt to identify those who did or did not report a current or past history of depression. About 4,000 women completed the screening phase; of those, a subgroup of women with ($n=332$) and without ($n=644$) a history of depression was enrolled in the prospective phase of the study and then followed with prospective assessments of serum hormone levels, menstrual characteristics, and standardized psychiatric evaluations. After more than 4 years of follow-up, the findings of this study demonstrated that women with a history of depression, assessed by a standardized psychiatric interview (the Structured Clinical Interview for DSM), are more likely to develop greater hormonal fluctuations in their serum levels of follicle-stimulating hormone (FSH), luteinizing hormone (LH), or estradiol over time, even while still being premenopausal. In addition, women with a history of depression are more likely to present with symptoms that characterize an earlier transition to menopause, including menstrual irregularities, hot flashes, and night sweats (Harlow et al. 1999).

A prospective study by Freeman et al. (2004) used mood and hormonal measures to assess 436 women, ages 35–47 years, during a 4-year period. They found an increased likelihood of depressive symptoms during the transition to menopause and a decreased likelihood after menopause, after adjusting for other predictors of depression. Hormonal associations provided corroborative evidence that the changing hormonal milieu contributes to dysphoric mood during the transition to menopause.

Epidemiologic studies have shown mixed results with respect to the association between depression and the menopausal transition (McKinlay 1996; Porter et al. 1996). One study (Maartens 2002) collected information from 2,103 women from Eindhoven, the Netherlands; the data obtained in 1994 (during a cross-sectional population survey) were compared with those obtained 3.5 years later (range: 2.8–4.7 years). The investigators used a cutoff score of 12 on the Edinburgh Depression Scale (EDS) to define presence of depression. By using multiple regression analyses, they demonstrated that the transition from pre- to perimenopause (mainly based on menstrual history) was significantly associated with a higher increase in EDS scores (odds ratio=1.8; 95% confidence interval, 1.1–3.3). Other independent factors contributing significantly to an increase in depressive symptoms over time included prior depression, financial problems, unemployment, transition from peri- to postmenopause, and death of a partner. If further confirmed, the findings derived from the Harvard Study of Moods and Cycles suggesting an association between depression and an earlier menopausal transition may result in significant public health implications, given the compound burden of illness. An earlier perimenopause would represent a prolonged exposure to a hypoestrogenic state, which has been associated with several medical conditions, such as loss of bone density, sexual dysfunction, decline in cognitive function, and a potential increased risk of cardiovascular disease. Also, there is substantial morbidity and economic burden inherent in the occurrence of depression. More recent findings derived from the Harvard Study of Moods and Cycles also suggest that women approaching menopause (i.e., presenting with irregular cycles and significant vasomotor symptoms) would be at significantly greater risk of developing depressive symptoms, even in the absence of prior episodes of depression (Soares 2003). This putative association could consolidate the view of an existing intrinsic connection between disrupted hormone milieu and brain functioning.

Despite evidence that hormonal fluctuations exert a psychological destabilizing action during certain reproductive cycle–related events, clinical trials have also demonstrated that sex hormones may in fact help to prevent or even treat depressive symptoms. This has already been shown in studies that examined the effects of treatment with estradiol for premenstrual depressive symptoms (Smith et al. 1995) and during the puerperium (Ahokas et al. 2001; Gregoire et al. 1996). It is noteworthy that these were mostly small studies, so further larger studies are needed to corroborate these promising findings. Double-blind, placebo-controlled studies have shown significant antidepressant benefit with the use of transdermal estradiol in perimenopausal women suffering from major depressive disorder, dysthymia, or minor depression (Schmidt et al. 2000; Soares et al. 2001a). Results obtained with the use of estradiol for postmenopausal depressed women were less promising (Cohen et al. 2003). Transdermal testosterone, however, has been shown to be efficacious for the treatment of psychological distress and decreased libido in some postmenopausal women (Shifren et al. 2000).

In this chapter, we examine the impact of sex hormones on brain functioning among peri- and postmenopausal women. Primarily, we review existing clinical data on the efficacy of several strategies, such as different hormone preparations and antidepressant augmentation, for the treatment of mood and cognitive disorders. The ultimate goal of any treatment strategy for women experiencing menopause-related symptoms is achieving a better quality of life.

The Menopausal Transition and Ovarian Changes

The mechanism by which neuroregulatory changes may occur during the transition to menopause is still largely unknown (Wise et al. 1996). Generally, one of the first detectable serum hormonal changes of perimenopause is a rising concentration of the pituitary gonadotropin FSH. The rising FSH concentration is probably caused by an exponential decline of gonadotropin-sensitive ovarian follicles as menopause approaches. Follicular development at this time has been demonstrated to be erratic, with consequent variability in estrogen levels and an increased percentage of anovulatory cycles (Shifren and Schiff 2000). Thus, the pituitary gland is stimulated to produce more FSH in an effort to stimulate the resistant follicles. The production of FSH and LH by the pituitary gland is subjected to a predominantly negative feedback by the ovarian sex steroids estrogen and progesterone. During perimenopause, there may be a fluctuation of circulating levels of sex steroids, particularly a reduction of estrogens and inhibins. The inhibins are gonadal peptides produced in the ovarian granulosa cells. The secretion of inhibin A generally follows that of estradiol and progesterone in the luteal phase of the menstrual cycle. Inhibin B is produced by nondominant ovarian follicles and is linked to the secretion of FSH to fine-tune the negative feedback system (North American Menopause Society 2000). Reproductive aging may occur as early as 10 years prior to menopause and is evidenced by a rising FSH level in the early follicular phase of the cycle and a decrease in inhibin B.

The fluctuation of both inhibin and estrogen may disturb the negative feedback on the pituitary FSH secretion, while LH production may remain in the normal range. However, serum levels of FSH and estrogens can fluctuate widely from cycle to cycle and from woman to woman during perimenopause. Consequently, confirmation of perimenopause is usually based on a woman's medical and menstrual history and, to a lesser extent, laboratory testing, as well as on the characteristics of reported somatic and emotional symptoms.

The perimenopause also interferes with the production and balance of different forms of estrogen present in women. The most biologically active form of estrogen is estradiol-17β, produced in the granulosa cells of the ovaries. In addition, both estradiol-17β and estrone, a less active form of estrogen, result from the conversion of testosterone and androstenedione by the enzyme aromatase (Adashi 1994). Estrone may also result from the peripheral aromatization of adrenal androstenedione, particularly in postmenopausal women (Shifren and Schiff 2000). Estriol, a very weak estrogen, is mostly produced during pregnancy by the placenta, and it can also be obtained by hepatic conversion of estrone.

The Menopausal Transition and Depression

The extent to which menopause is associated with specific psychiatric disorders, particularly mood disorders, continues to be a controversial topic (Schmidt et al. 1997; Stone and Pearlstein 1994). Contemporary epidemiologic studies have failed to substantiate that mood disorders are more common in naturally menopausal women than in younger women (McKinlay 1996; Porter et al. 1996). Most studies examining this question vary greatly in design (Burt et al. 1998; Soares and Cohen 2001). For example, data are derived from different settings (gynecologic clinics, community-based studies) and have included women with diverse menopausal status, ascertained primarily by age. These studies also suffer from a lack of standardized instruments to evaluate psychiatric symptoms (Bungay et al. 1980; Jaszmann et al. 1969).

It appears that women who attend gynecologic menopause clinics differ from menopausal women in community settings. For example, the likelihood of experiencing a depressive disorder during the perimenopausal period is higher in women attending menopause clinics than in community women in this age group (Anderson et al. 1987; Hay et al. 1994). However, it has been speculated that women who seek treatment for menopause-related symptoms through specialized gynecologic clinics may not be representative of the population of perimenopausal women overall but rather represent a subgroup with a high prevalence of physical and emotional symptoms, including depressive disorders (Burt et al. 1998; Schmidt et al. 1997). Most cross-sectional studies suggest that perimenopausal women (commonly defined as women ages 45–55 years with changes in their menstrual pattern) are more likely to report depressive symptoms compared with premenopausal women (those of the same age who still have regular menstrual periods) or postmenopausal women (Avis and McKinlay 1995; Kaufert et al. 1992). A study of more than 500 pre-, peri-, and postmenopausal women in a primary care clinic demonstrated that marital disruption and unemployment, as well as somatic symptoms and past history of depression, may influence the likelihood of depressive symptoms in this population, regardless of menopausal status. The presence of severe hot flashes, however, was a risk factor for depression only among the perimenopausal women, even though hot flashes occurred in all three menopausal groups (Joffe et al. 2002). Depressive disorders appear to be highly prevalent among women with surgically induced menopause, compared with naturally menopausal women (McKinlay et al. 1987). One possible explanation is that women with nonspecific complaints and unrecognized mood and anxiety disorders would tend to attribute these complaints to altered reproductive hormones. They would seek somatic treatment more often than psychological help and then be more inclined to accept undergoing hysterectomy and oophorectomy among the treatments to alleviate such symptoms.

Various psychosocial theories attempt to explain the mechanism of mood changes seen in some women during perimenopause, some of which are reviewed in different chapters of this book. One of the physiological theories used to explain the occurrence of depressive symptoms is called the *domino theory* (Campbell and Whitehead 1977). This theory proposes that the discomfort caused by night sweats and hot flashes provokes physical changes (sleep disturbance) and, consequently, affects mood stability. Hence, investigators have speculated that the capacity of estrogen to improve mood is secondary to relief of somatic menopausal symptoms and normalization of sleep. The *estrogen withdrawal theory* (Schmidt et al. 1997), however, proposes that the onset or worsening of mood symptoms in perimenopausal women results from a significant decline in peripheral concentrations of estrogen. However, it has been established that estrogen levels may increase during the early perimenopausal period and then drop again, which would contradict the estrogen withdrawal theory (Burger et al. 1995). As a higher incidence of depression can be observed in women who have undergone bilateral oophorectomy (surgical menopause) compared with that observed among naturally menopausal women, it is unquestionable that abrupt changes in estrogen levels play some role in the development of depressive symptoms in this subpopulation (Schmidt et al. 1997).

Sex Hormones, the Central Nervous System, and the Treatment of Depression and Cognitive Deficits

Estrogen

It is not fully understood how estrogen works in the brain (Fink et al. 1996). However, understanding of the interactions between estrogens and brain functioning has increased over the last decade (Joffe and Cohen 1998). The distribution of various estradiol receptors (named estradiol-17α and estradiol-17β receptors, to date) in different brain regions (such as the medial amygdala, hippocampus, and limbic system) and their distinct up- or downregulation by estradiol contribute to the complexity of estrogen's effects on the central nervous system (Genazzani et al. 1997; Maggi and Perez 1985; Silva et al. 2001; Woolley 1999). It has been speculated that estrogens interact with membrane and nuclear receptors. Estrogens act through nuclear receptors as transcription factors by binding as dimers to specific response elements in DNA and regulating the expression of targeted genes. In addition, the effects of estrogens on membrane receptors possibly modulate the synthesis, release, and metabolism of monoamines. Estrogens may also up- or downregulate the excitability of neurons quite rapidly, probably acting through G-protein–dependent mechanisms (McEwen and Alves 1999; Stahl 2001). Estrogens exert an agonist effect on serotonergic activity by increasing the number of serotonergic receptors and the transport and uptake of the neurotransmitter; estrogens also increase the synthesis of serotonin, upregulate 5-hydroxytryptamine 1 (5-HT_1) receptors, downregulate 5-HT_2 receptors, and decrease monoamine oxidase activity (Halbreich and Kahn 2001). Estrogens appear to increase noradrenergic (NA) activity by increasing NA turnover and decreasing NA reuptake, and by decreasing the number and sensitivity of dopamine D_2 receptors (Garlow et al. 1999). Last, estrogens induce new dendritic spine formation and synapses in hippocampal neurons, and they regulate neurotropic factors and neuropeptides, such as neuropeptide Y and corticotropin-releasing factor. This may explain the putative impact of estrogens on the thermoregulatory system and their effects on voracity or appetite and blood pressure. Estrogen availability may also modulate the binding affinity of 5-HT receptors, as shown in animal models (Bethea et al. 2002) and in neuroimaging clinical studies (Kugaya et al. 2003).

Despite clinical and laboratory evidence of putative antidepressant benefit of estrogen use for menopausal women, some conflicting results can be found in the literature, possibly because of multiple factors, such as the heterogeneity of methods to define and assess menopausal and hormonal status, the lack of control with respect to the occurrence and severity of vasomotor symptoms, the lack of standardized diagnostic and outcome measures, the differences in hormone preparations, and the wide range of doses and methods of administration (Holte 1998).

Estrogens are available in many preparations, including transdermal patches and creams, oral tablets, intranasal or sublingual formulations, injections, and subdermal implants (Ramachandran and Fleisher 2000; Stahl 2001). Most data on the efficacy and safety of estrogens in the United States have been based on studies using oral conjugated estrogens. Differences in the pharmacokinetic aspects of estrogen preparations may contribute to the lack of consistency across the studies regarding the effect of estrogen treatment on mood (Halbreich and Kahn 2001). Existing data suggest that transdermal administration of estradiol (matrix-type system) avoids the first-pass circulation through the liver and gastrointestinal absorption and therefore provides a rapid rise in the serum concentration of estradiol and nearly constant serum levels (i.e., constant estradiol-to-estrone ratios) over the entire application period, particularly in postmenopausal women (Ramachandran and Fleischer 2000; Scott et al. 1991). It is interesting that treatment studies of transdermal estradiol for premenstrual syndrome (PMS) (100 µg/day vs. 200 µg/day) (Smith et al. 1995), puerperal depression (randomized placebo-controlled study, 200 µg/day) (Gregoire et al. 1996), and perimenopausal depression (randomized placebo-controlled studies, 50 µg/day or 100 µg/day) (Schmidt et al. 2000; Soares et al. 2001a) have shown positive results. Oral estrogens, however, are metabolized through the hepatic portal system, which results in higher conversion to a less active metabolite (estrone) and consequently lower bioavailability of estradiol (Fraser and Wang 1998). Most estrogen trials that failed to detect an antidepressant efficacy in comparison with placebo used either oral preparations of conjugated equine estrogen or piperazine sulfate estrone (Coope et al. 1975; Strickler et al. 1977; Thompson and Oswald 1977).

The use of transdermal estradiol (0.05 mg/day) showed superior efficacy compared with placebo in 34 perimenopausal women with major and minor depression, in the presence or absence of hot flashes (Schmidt et al. 2000). These findings corroborate the idea that the effects of estrogen on mood and on vasomotor symptoms, the latter possibly resulting from hypothalamic thermoregulatory dysfunction, are independent. Similar results were found in a larger sample of perimenopausal women suffering from depressive disorders (mostly major depression) treated with transdermal estradiol (0.1 mg/day) or placebo (Soares et al. 2001a). In this study, most women were able to sustain an antidepressant benefit after a 4-week washout period, despite the reemergence of vasomotor symptoms, again suggesting the existence of independent effects of estradiol on mood and vasomotor symptoms.

Studies on postmenopausal subpopulations have shown less compelling evidence of estrogen's antidepressant efficacy. Negative results have been reported when conjugated estrogen (George et al. 1973) or estrogen sulfate (Coppen et al. 1977) were given to surgically induced menopausal women. In addition, the use of transdermal estradiol (50 µg/day) in postmenopausal women did not show superior efficacy when compared with placebo for the treatment of depressive symptoms (Saletu et al. 1995). Antidepressant benefit of estrogen for postmenopausal women appears to be limited even when examined in open clinical trials (Cohen et al. 2003). It is possible that postmenopausal women would require a higher dose and prolonged treatment with estradiol to obtain a satisfactory antidepressant response to estrogen treatment, possibly because of the altered sensitivity of their estrogen receptors. Also, it is possible that perimenopausal depressed women are uniquely responsive to the mood-enhancing effects of estradiol.

Studies attempting to show the efficacy of estrogen as an adjunctive therapy for major depression in postmenopausal women have had mixed results, possibly as a result of methodologic limitations. Retrospective analyses of older women treated with fluoxetine (Amsterdam et al. 1999; Schneider et al. 1997) with or without hormone therapy (HT) have shown greater improvement in depressive symptoms among those who received fluoxetine plus HT than among those receiving the antidepressant alone. However, in these studies women were not randomly assigned to HT, which might have contributed to a selection bias. A pooled analysis of women treated with venlafaxine with or without concomitant use of HT for depression found no evidence suggesting a significant change in efficacy associated with HT use (Entsuah et al. 2001). However, the concomitant use of HT could maximize some of the benefits obtained with selective serotonin reuptake inhibitors in perimenopausal women, particularly in promoting greater well-being (Soares et al. 2003).

There is some evidence that estrogen enhances learning and memory in older women, although the data are mixed (Barrett-Connor and Kritz-Silverstein 1993; Szklo et al. 1996). Some studies have found that estrogen enhances memory in women with Alzheimer's disease (Henderson et al. 1996) and may have a protective effect against the development of some dementias (LeBlanc et al. 2001; Maki et al. 2001; Paganini-Hill and Henderson 1996; Resnick et al. 1997; Sherwin 1999; Smith et al. 2001). A comparison of cognitive performance in normal postmenopausal women versus those on HT found that those on estrogen had superior cognitive skills (Yaffe et al. 1998b), further supporting this hypothesis (Wickelgren 1997). However, an interim analysis from the Framingham Heart Study in Boston, based on a large population-based nested case-control study, showed that the use of estrogen therapy in menopausal women was not associated with a reduced risk of developing Alzheimer's disease (Seshadri et al. 2001).

The Women's Health Initiative (WHI) Study, a randomized, controlled, primary prevention trial (planned duration: 8.5 years), randomly assigned 16,608 postmenopausal women ages 50–79 years (mean age: 63) with an intact uterus at baseline to receive estrogen plus progestin (0.625 mg of conjugated equine estrogen [CEE] plus 2.5 mg of medroxyprogesterone acetate [MPA]; $n=8,506$) or placebo ($n=8,102$). The primary outcome measure was coronary heart disease, with invasive breast cancer as the primary adverse outcome. Other measures included cases of stroke, pulmonary embolism, endometrial cancer, colorectal cancer, and hip fracture. In May 2002, after a mean of 5.2 years of follow-up, the trial was stopped by recommendation of the data- and safety-monitoring board because the overall health risks associated with combined estrogen plus progestin had exceeded the benefits (mainly, more strokes, coronary heart disease, invasive breast cancer, and pulmonary embolisms per 10,000 person-years; Rossouw et al. 2002). In February 2004, the study using estrogen alone (or placebo), including postmenopausal women with hysterectomy, was also stopped because the burden of incident disease events was similar in the estrogen-alone and placebo groups—and therefore estrogen alone would not result in any significant benefit (Anderson et al. 2004). Last, although not specifically designed to examine the benefits of HT for psychological symptoms, mood, or cognition, the WHI Study also reported the impact of estrogen (plus progestin) on quality of life, including questions on general health, vitality, mental health, depressive symptoms, and sexual satisfaction. At 3 years, there were no significant benefits in terms of any quality-of-life outcomes (Hays et al. 2003).

A subgroup of women age 65 years or older was evaluated to assess the incidence of probable dementia (primary outcome) and mild cognitive impairment (secondary outcome) in the WHI Memory Study. After a mean time of 4 years postrandomization, there was an increased risk of probable dementia observed among those using estrogen plus progestin, as compared with placebo (Shumaker et al. 2003). In addition, the study was not able to identify a significant improvement in cognitive function among hormone users, as compared with placebo (Rapp et al. 2003).

The clinical implications of the main findings derived from the WHI Study, as well as some comments on its study limitations, are further discussed later in this chapter.

Effects of Progesterone on the Central Nervous System

Progesterone receptors can be found in many of the same brain areas as estrogen receptors, such as the limbic system and the hypothalamus (Sherwin 1999). Progesterone appears to have a negative effect on mood, mainly as a result of the occurrence of increased irritability and dysphoria; however, hypnotic, anxiolytic, and antiepileptic effects have been described with its use (Halbreich 1997; Lawrie et al. 1998). Animal studies suggest the existence of a potent dose-dependent modulation of progesterone's metabolites—allopregnenolone and pregnenolone—on the γ-aminobutyric acid (GABA) A receptor, enhancing GABAergic inhibitory neurotransmission (Freeman et al. 1993).

The impact of progesterone on mood has been more systematically studied among women suffering from PMS and premenstrual dysphoric disorder. Randomized, placebo-controlled studies utilizing either progesterone suppositories, administered vaginally or rectally, or oral progesterone have shown mixed results. In a systematic review of 14 trials in which progesterone preparations were compared with placebo for the treatment of women with PMS, Wyatt and colleagues (2001) did not find evidence to support the use of progesterone or progestogens for the management of premenstrual complaints.

To examine the effect of progesterone on mood in postmenopausal women, de Wit et al. (2001) administered weekly intramuscular injections of progesterone (25 mg, 50 mg, or 100 mg) to postmenopausal women for 1 month. In the same study, premenopausal women with regular menstrual cycles received 100 mg of intramuscular progesterone weekly. The progesterone caused slight sedation among postmenopausal women who received the highest dose of progesterone. Premenopausal women, however, experienced mild sedative effects despite receiving supraphysiologic doses of progesterone. In addition, serum levels of progesterone metabolites (allopregnenolone) did not correlate with mood symptoms. Less is known with regard to effects of synthetic progestins—commonly used in clinical practice—on brain function, although it has been speculated that their metabolites have lower potency than allopregnenolone (Wihlback et al. 2001). Studies of the contraceptive depot-MPA and mood have shown mixed results. Most prospective studies have shown either no effect of depot-MPA on mood or a minimal increase in negative mood symptoms (Gupta et al. 2001; Westhoff et al. 1995; Wieland et al. 1997). Civic and colleagues (2000) compared depressive symptoms in users and nonusers of depot-MPA. Continuous users of depot-MPA reported more depressive symptoms than nonusers.

Androgens

The neuroprotective properties of androgens (Wolf and Kirschbaum 1999), as well as their essential role in the organization or programming of brain circuits (Rubinow and Schmidt 1996), are supported by animal studies and considerable clinical evidence. Androgens are produced in women by the adrenal glands and ovaries, and include testosterone, androstenedione, dehydroepiandrosterone (DHEA), and dehydroepiandrosterone sulfate (DHEA-S). The last two, DHEA and DHEA-S, are adrenal steroids, available in higher concentrations than other androgens (Morrison 1997). Circulating levels of androgens decrease significantly with aging, as a result of decreased adrenal production and a reduction in midcycle ovarian secretion (Davis

1999; Zumoff and Bradlow 1980). Premenopausal women produce 300 μg of testosterone per day, originating from both adrenal and ovarian secretion. If a woman has received bilateral oophorectomy, testosterone and androstenedione production will be limited to 50% (Morley 2001). Reduction in androgen levels also result in decreased production of estrogens in extragonadal tissues.

Testosterone

The impact of testosterone on mood and behavior in women has been well described. Accumulating data suggest an association between serum levels of testosterone and traits of aggressive behavior (Archer 1991; Christiansen 1993). Levels of androgens (total testosterone, free testosterone, and androstenedione) have been correlated with some aspects of sexuality in the female population (Cashdan 1995). Plasma testosterone levels are high around the time of ovulation; hence, several studies have aimed to identify evidence of an androgenic enhancement of sexual behavior at this time (Shifren and Schiff 2000).

Depressive symptoms and anxiety, as well as decreased libido, have been described among postmenopausal women who present with decreased testosterone, particularly after oophorectomy. Testosterone supplementation has been shown to alleviate these symptoms (Sherwin and Gelfand 1985). Shifren and colleagues (2000) examined the impact of transdermal testosterone in 75 women (ages 31–56) who underwent hysterectomy and oophorectomy. They received patches containing 150 or 300 μg of testosterone or placebo for 12 weeks. All subjects received concomitant treatment with oral conjugated estrogens. When compared with placebo, women who received testosterone reported greater psychological well-being and a significant improvement in mood and anxiety. They also reported a qualitative improvement in their sexual life. Treatment with testosterone was well tolerated, without significant occurrence of acne or hirsutism.

Dehydroepiandrosterone and Its Sulfate

Dehydroepiandrosterone and its sulfate may have a modulatory effect on mood. Barrett-Connor and colleagues (1999) examined 699 women (ages 50–89) in a community-based sample and tried to establish a significant association between depressive symptoms and serum concentrations of gonadal steroids. Only DHEA and DHEA-S levels were found to have an inverse correlation with the presence of depressive symptoms. Another study of 394 older women (more than 65 years of age) showed similar results. The modulatory effect of DHEA on mood may be explained by several mechanisms: its partial biotransformation into testosterone and estrogens (both presumably with positive effects on mood), its effects on GABA receptors and cortisol, and an increase in serotonergic activity in the brain (Yaffe et al. 1998a).

The antidepressant benefit obtained with DHEA has been documented in placebo-controlled trials. Wolkowitz et al. (1997) administered oral DHEA (30–90 mg/day) or placebo to 22 patients (10 women) for 6 weeks. In contrast with those who received placebo, subjects who were given DHEA experienced significant improvement in mood, with good treatment tolerability and no gender differences regarding efficacy. Further studies would help to delineate the therapeutic role of DHEA for women with depression, particularly long-term benefits compared with adverse events, and potential risks associated with effects on hormone-sensitive tumors.

Use of Hormone Treatments in the Post–Women's Health Initiative Era

For many decades, women and health professionals were taught about the benefits and risks of HT. Essentially, HT had been administered to alleviate physical symptoms associated with the menopausal transition (short-term use of HT) and to help in preventing the clinical consequences of an estrogen-deficient state, including osteoporosis and cardiovascular disease (long-term use of HT). More recently, the list of benefits of short-term HT was expanded, incorporating preliminary but promising findings on mood and cognition. Nonetheless, results from large prospective studies were highly desired, because they could provide more robust information on the risks and benefits of long-term HT.

The results from the WHI Study have caused both disappointment and apprehension. The impact of HT on well-being and sexual satisfaction was not significant. In addition, in a subgroup of subjects in whom a higher risk of developing dementia had been identified (in the WHI Memory Study), HT failed to prevent the development of cognitive deficits. As a first reaction, physicians and patients felt betrayed, and many have decided to discontinue their HT regimens. Still others who did not abandon their prescription hormones are now questioning their current treatment and potential alternatives. Most women and their doctors are now facing a difficult situation: How should they deal with menopause-related physical and emotional symptoms? Is there a role for HT in the post-WHI era? See Chapter 6, Medical Aspects of Perimenopause and Menopause, and Chapter 7, Gynecologic Aspects of Perimenopause and Menopause, for further discussion of WHI results.

The results from the WHI Study should be carefully interpreted. In fact, various menopause societies have expressed their concerns, and investigators and seasoned clinicians have pointed out that some of these results were a "direct consequence of unsuitable population selection (e.g., older, postmenopausal women), terribly wide inclusion criteria (e.g., subjects with various preexisting medical conditions), lack of adequate assessments (e.g., lack of adequate assessment for menopause-related somatic symptoms), and the incongruous treatment choice (CEE+MPA)" (Notelovitz 2003, p. 8). The main criticism, however, should be focused on the misinterpretation and generalization of the WHI data; this study was designed essentially to examine the impact of a specific hormone formulation (CEE+MPA) on the relative risk of developing cardiovascular disease, cancer, or fractures in older, postmenopausal women. The study was *not* designed to address the impact or safety of using CEE+MPA (or any other hormone preparation) for the management of younger, perimenopausal women with menopause-related somatic and psychological complaints—for example, for the treatment of hot flashes and depressive symptoms. Unfortunately, such a distinction has not always been made by the lay press or even addressed clearly in discussions among physicians or between them and their patients.

The benefits and safety of long-term use of conjugated estrogens and medroxyprogesterone are now in question; research will undoubtedly increase in the search for safer alternatives, such as selective estrogen receptor modulators and diet supplementation, for prevention of menopause-related conditions. However, clinicians and health professionals should continue considering many factors when advising women who are approaching menopause or are postmenopausal on treatment choices. For example, it has been speculated that for those currently on HT, an abrupt treatment discontinuation could lead to the occurrence or reemergence of somatic symptoms, interfering with sleep patterns, physical well-being, and most probably mood; more research is needed to examine whether a gradual treatment discontinuation could decrease the risk of mood instability, anxiety, and insomnia, especially in women with a past history of these symptoms.

There are many HT preparations available, including other types of estrogens and progestins (e.g., estradiol-17β, micronized progesterone). The WHI Study has yielded data only on the use of conjugated estrogens and medroxyprogesterone; long-term data on other HT regimens are sparse, and certainly overdue. As already seen with various antidepressants, HTs differ with respect to absorption, metabolism, and bioavailability. It has been suggested, for example, that estradiol provides a more positive effect on mood and cognition and could offer a different risk-benefit profile, given its similarity to endogenous sex hormones (Ramachandran and Fleisher 2000). Nonetheless, in the absence of more data, we cannot ensure the safety of switching patients to another hormone combination. In fact, current U.S. Food and Drug Administration guidelines recommend that in the absence of data on other hormone preparations and different dosages, the risks should be assumed to be similar. The use of estrogens plus progestins is not recommended for prevention of cardiovascular disease. This hormone preparation should be used "at the lowest effective doses, and for the shortest duration consistent with treatment goals and risks for the individual woman" (U.S. Food and Drug Administration 2004).

Ongoing studies suggest that hormone interventions (including testosterone and DHEA) may play an important role in promoting well-being among aging men and women. More than ever, it is imperative to better delineate their clinical indications and to learn more about risks and benefits associated with different hormone preparations before they enter widespread population use.

Selective Estrogen Receptor Modulators and Their Impact on Mood and Cognition

Selective estrogen receptor modulators (SERMs) are synthetic, nonhormonal compounds that act as estrogen agonists on some organs in the body and estrogen antagonists on other organs. SERMs may have estrogen antagonist effects on breast tissue and estrogen agonist effects on the cardiovascular system and bone (Mayeux 2001) but differ in their effects on other body organs (Genazzani et al. 1997, 1999). The use of SERMs such as tamoxifen has become an important tool as an adjuvant therapy for breast cancer patients. Such use might result in an increased occurrence of symptoms in breast cancer patients similar to those symptoms observed in menopause, such as hot flashes and night sweats, and contribute to a poorer quality of life. For example, evidence suggests that the estrogen receptors that mediate the stimulatory effect on the serotonergic system might be blocked by tamoxifen (Sumner et al. 1999; Wissink et al. 2001). Tamoxifen may also block the neuroprotective effects of estradiol by downregulating neurotransmitter activity (Thompson et al. 1999). It is reasonable to believe that tamoxifen would have a depressive effect on mood as a result of this antiestrogen effect on the neuroendocrine system. However, the data on this depressive effect have been conflicting. There were no significant differences between the effects caused by placebo or tamoxifen on depression (based on Center for Epidemiologic Studies Depression Scale scores) and quality of life (assessed by the SF-36 questionnaire) in the Breast Cancer Prevention Trial (Fisher et al. 1998). This trial included 13,388 women ages 35–60 years who were at an increased risk for breast cancer. A smaller trial ($N=257$) found an increase in depression among women who were receiving tamoxifen (23 of 155, or 15%) after completing initial treatment for breast cancer, compared with women who did not receive tamoxifen (3 of 102, or 3%). In some cases, the depression required discontinuing therapy with tamoxifen (Cathcart et al. 1993). It has been speculated that women experiencing depression while using tamoxifen would have such mood changes as a function of developing hot flashes, night sweats, and increased vaginal discharge. Observational studies, however, have not shown a negative impact on quality of life (Ganz 2001).

Less is known about the neuroendocrine effects of raloxifene hydrochloride, a SERM used to treat osteoporosis but also being investigated for its putative benefits in breast cancer prevention. A finding reported from the Multiple Outcomes of Raloxifene Evaluation trial—a multicenter, randomized clinical trial of raloxifene versus placebo—showed no overall difference in cognitive functioning between postmenopausal women assigned to receive 60 mg of raloxifene or placebo (Yaffe et al. 2001). This study also showed a trend toward a slower decline in verbal memory among raloxifene users, corroborating other findings (Nickelsen et al. 1999). Improvement in some domains of quality of life were found in a multicenter, double-blind clinical trial of 398 women randomly assigned to one of four groups: raloxifene 60 mg ($n=97$), raloxifene 150 mg ($n=100$), CEEs 0.625 mg ($n=96$), or placebo ($n=105$). Anxiety or fears scores improved in the raloxifene group regardless of baseline estradiol levels, previous hormone use, or years of postmenopause (Strickler et al. 2000). Jarkova and colleagues (2002) examined a group of nondepressed postmenopausal women receiving 60 mg of raloxifene ($n=18$) or placebo ($n=18$) to investigate the effect of raloxifene on mood (assessed by changes in Hamilton Rating Scale for Depression scores). The findings suggest that raloxifene does not negatively influence mood in a nondepressed, younger postmenopausal population. A larger study of *depressed* menopausal women is necessary to determine a potential mood improvement effect of raloxifene.

Conclusive statements cannot be made concerning the potential depressive or cognitive effects of SERMs at this time. Though there is some evidence that SERMs block the serotonergic modulation exerted by estradiol in animal models (Genazzani et al. 1997), it is unclear to what extent its clinical use may affect mood or cognitive function. See Chapter 6 and Chapter 7 for further information about SERMS.

Conclusion

Accumulating evidence suggests intrinsic and complex interactions between sex hormones and brain functioning. Naturally, there are many factors that might play an important role in the development of depressive symptoms and cognitive deficits in women.

The extent to which the use of estrogen, testosterone, or DHEA may help to improve treatment outcomes among women who present with depressive symptoms or cognitive decline is still unclear, given the methodologic limitations of the existing data. Antidepressants, mood stabilizers, and psychotherapy will continue to be well-established treatments for mood disturbances. Other treatments have been sought for alleviation of cognitive decline in the aging population. However, it is plausible that subgroups of menopausal women will benefit from the combined use of hormonal and nonhormonal strategies.

The search for an improved quality of life for our female patients will certainly stimulate further studies to define strategies to ameliorate depressive symptoms and cognitive deficits, with efficacy and safety and with fewer side effects. Psychiatrists and other health professionals involved in psychiatric care should therefore be aware of the accumulating data on the psychotropic effects of sex hormones to better treat these subpopulations.

References

Adashi EY: The climacteric ovary as a functional gonadotropin-driven androgen-producing gland. Fertil Steril 62:20–27, 1994

Ahokas A, Kaukoranta J, Wahlbeck K, et al: Estrogen deficiency in severe postpartum depression: successful treatment with sublingual physiologic 17beta-estradiol: a preliminary study. J Clin Psychiatry 62:332–336, 2001

Amsterdam J, Garcia-Espana F, Fawcett J, et al: Fluoxetine efficacy in menopausal women with and without estrogen replacement. J Affect Disord 55:11–17, 1999

Anderson E, Hamburger S, Liu JH, et al: Characteristics of menopausal women seeking assistance. Am J Obstet Gynecol 156:428–433, 1987

Anderson GL, Limacher M, Assaf AR, et al: Effects of conjugated equine estrogen in postmenopausal women with hysterectomy: the Women's Health Initiative randomized controlled trial. JAMA 291:1701–1712, 2004

Archer J: The influence of testosterone on human aggression. Br J Psychol 82:1–28, 1991

Avis NE, McKinlay SM: The Massachusetts Women's Health Study: an epidemiologic investigation of the menopause. JAMA 50:5–49, 63, 1995

Barrett-Connor E, Kritz-Silverstein D: Estrogen replacement therapy and cognitive function in older women. JAMA 269:2637–2641, 1993

Barrett-Connor E, von Muhlen D, Laughlin GA, et al: Endogenous levels of dehydroepiandrosterone sulfate, but not other sex hormones, are associated with depressed mood in older women: the Rancho Bernardo Study. J Am Geriatr Soc 47:685–691, 1999

Bethea CL, Lu NZ, Gundlah C, et al: Diverse actions of ovarian steroids in the sero-
    tonin neural system. Front Neuroendocrinol 23:41–100, 2002
Born L, Steiner M: The relationship between menarche and depression in adoles-
    cence. CNS Spectr 6:126–138, 2001
Bungay GT, Vessey MP, McPherson CK: Study of symptoms in middle life with spe-
    cial reference to the menopause. Br Med J 281:181–183, 1980
Burger HG, Dudley EC, Hopper JL, et al: The endocrinology of the menopausal tran-
    sition: a cross-sectional study of a population-based sample. J Clin Endocrinol
    Metab 80:3537–3545, 1995
Burt VK, Altshuler LL, Rasgon N: Depressive symptoms in the perimenopause: prev-
    alence, assessment, and guidelines for treatment. Harv Rev Psychiatry 6:121–
    132, 1998
Campbell S, Whitehead M: Oestrogen therapy and the menopausal syndrome. Clin
    Obstet Gynaecol 4:31–47, 1977
Cashdan E: Hormones, sex, and status in women. Horm Behav 29:354–366, 1995
Cathcart CK, Jones SE, Pumroy CS, et al: Clinical recognition and management of
    depression in node negative breast cancer patients treated with tamoxifen.
    Breast Cancer Res Treat 27:277–281, 1993
Christiansen K: Behavioural effects of androgen in men and women. J Endocrinol
    170:39–48, 1993
Civic D, Scholes D, Ichikawa L, et al: Depressive symptoms in users and nonusers of
    depot medroxyprogesterone acetate. Contraception 61:385–390, 2000
Cohen LS, Soares CN, Poitras JR, et al: Short-term use of estradiol for depression in
    perimenopausal and postmenopausal women: a preliminary report. Am J Psy-
    chiatry 160:1519–1522, 2003
Coope J, Thomson JM, Poller L: Effects of "natural oestrogen" replacement therapy
    on menopausal symptoms and blood clotting. Br Med J 4:139–143, 1975
Coppen A, Bishop M, Beard R: Effects of piperazine oestrone sulphate on plasma
    tryptophan, oestrogens, gonadotrophins and psychological functioning in
    women following hysterectomy. Curr Med Res Opin 4:29–36, 1977
Davis S: The therapeutic use of androgens in women. J Steroid Biochem Mol Biol
    69:177–184, 1999
de Wit H, Schmitt L, Purdy R, et al: Effects of acute progesterone administration in
    healthy postmenopausal women and normally cycling women. Psychoneuroen-
    docrinology 26:697–710, 2001
Entsuah AR, Huang H, Thase ME: Response and remission rates in different subpop-
    ulations with major depressive disorder administered venlafaxine, selective se-
    rotonin reuptake inhibitors, or placebo. J Clin Psychiatry 62:869–877, 2001
Fink G, Sumner BE, Rosie R, et al: Estrogen control of central neurotransmission: ef-
    fect on mood, mental state, and memory. Cell Mol Neurobiol 16:325–344, 1996
Fisher B, Costantino JP, Wickerham DL, et al: Tamoxifen for prevention of breast can-
    cer: report of the National Surgical Adjuvant Breast and Bowel Project P-1 Study.
    J Natl Cancer Inst 90:1371–1388, 1998

Fraser I, Wang Y: New delivery systems for hormone replacement therapy, in The Management of Menopause—Annual Book Review. Edited by Studd J. London, Parthenon, 1998, pp 101–110

Freeman EW, Purdy RH, Coutifaris C, et al: Anxiolytic metabolites of progesterone: correlation with mood and performance measures following oral progesterone administration to healthy female volunteers. Neuroendocrinology 58:478–484, 1993

Freeman EW, Sammel MD, Liu L, et al: Hormones and menopausal status as predictors of depression in women in transition to menopause. Arch Gen Psychiatry 61:62–70, 2004

Ganz PA: Impact of tamoxifen adjuvant therapy on symptoms, functioning, and quality of life. J Natl Cancer Inst Monogr 30:130–134, 2001

Garlow S, Musselman D, Nemeroff C: The neurochemistry of mood disorders: clinical studies, in Neurobiology of Mental Illness. Edited by Charney D, Nestler E, Bunney B. New York, Oxford University Press, 1999, pp 348–364

Genazzani AR, Lucchesi A, Stomati M, et al: Effects of sex steroid hormones on the neuroendocrine system. Eur J Contracep Reprod Health Care 2:63–69, 1997

Genazzani AR, Bernardi F, Stomati M, et al: Raloxifene analog LY 117018 effects on central and peripheral beta-endorphin. Gynecol Endocrinol 13:249–258, 1999

George GC, Utian WH, Beaumont PJ, et al: Effect of exogenous oestrogens on minor psychiatric symptoms in postmenopausal women. S Afr Med J 47:2387–2388, 1973

Gregoire AJ, Kumar R, Everitt B, et al: Transdermal oestrogen for treatment of severe postnatal depression. Lancet 347:930–933, 1996

Gupta N, O'Brien R, Jacobsen LJ, et al: Mood changes in adolescents using depot-medroxyprogesterone acetate for contraception: a prospective study. J Pediatr Adolesc Gynecol 14:71–76, 2001

Halbreich U: Hormonal interventions with psychopharmacological potential: an overview. Psychopharmacol Bull 33:281–286, 1997

Halbreich U, Kahn LS: Role of estrogen in the aetiology and treatment of mood disorders. CNS Drugs 15:797–817, 2001

Harlow BL, Cohen LS, Otto MW, et al: Prevalence and predictors of depressive symptoms in older premenopausal women: the Harvard Study of Moods and Cycles. Arch Gen Psychiatry 56:418–424, 1999

Harlow BL, Wise LA, Otto MW, et al: Depression and its influence on reproductive endocrine and menstrual cycle markers associated with perimenopause: the Harvard Study of Moods and Cycles. Arch Gen Psychiatry 60:29–36, 2003

Hay AG, Bancroft J, Johnstone EC: Affective symptoms in women attending a menopause clinic. Br J Psychiatry 164:513–516, 1994

Hays J, Ockene JK, Brunner RL, et al: Effects of estrogen plus progestin on health-related quality of life. N Engl J Med 348:1839–1854, 2003

Henderson VW, Watt L, Buckwalter JG: Cognitive skills associated with estrogen replacement in women with Alzheimer's disease. Psychoneuroendocrinology 21:421–430, 1996

Holte A: Menopause, mood and hormone replacement therapy: methodological issues. Maturitas 29:5–18, 1998

Jarkova NB, Martenyi F, Masanauskaite D, et al: Mood effect of raloxifene in postmenopausal women. Maturitas 42:71–75, 2002

Jaszmann L, van Lith ND, Zaat JCA: The perimenopausal symptoms: the statistical analysis of a survey: part A. Med Gynaecol Sociol 4:268–277, 1969

Joffe H, Cohen LS: Estrogen, serotonin, and mood disturbance: where is the therapeutic bridge? Biol Psychiatry 44:798–811, 1998

Joffe H, Hennen J, Soares CN, et al: Hot flushes associated with depression in perimenopausal women seeking primary care. Menopause 9:392–398, 2002

Kaufert PA, Gilbert P, Tate R: The Manitoba Project: a re-examination of the link between menopause and depression. Maturitas 14:143–155, 1992

Kessler RC, McGonagle KA, Zhao S, et al: Lifetime and 12-month prevalence of DSM-III-R psychiatric disorders in the United States. Results from the National Comorbidity Survey. Arch Gen Psychiatry 51:8–19, 1994

Kugaya A, Epperson CN, Zoghbi S, et al: Increase in prefrontal cortex serotonin 2A receptors following estrogen treatment in postmenopausal women. Am J Psychiatry 160:1522–1524, 2003

Lawrie TA, Hofmeyr GJ, De Jager M, et al: A double-blind randomised placebo-controlled trial of postnatal norethisterone enanthate: the effect on postnatal depression and serum hormones. Br J Obstet Gynaecol 105:1082–1090, 1998

LeBlanc ES, Janowsky J, Chan BK, et al: Hormone replacement therapy and cognition: systematic review and meta-analysis. JAMA 285:1489–1499, 2001

Maartens LW, Knottnerus JA, Pop VJ: Menopausal transition and increased depressive symptomatology: a community-based prospective study. Maturitas 42:195–200, 2002

Maggi A, Perez J: Role of female gonadal hormones in the CNS: clinical and experimental aspects. Life Sci 37:893–906, 1985

Maki P, Zonderman A, Resnick S: Enhanced verbal memory in nondemented elderly women receiving hormone-replacement therapy. Am J Psychiatry 158:227–233, 2001

Mayeux R: Can estrogen or selective estrogen-receptor modulators preserve cognitive function in elderly women? N Engl J Med 344:1242–1244, 2001

McEwen BS, Alves SE: Estrogen actions in the central nervous system. Endocr Rev 20:279–307, 1999

McKinlay JB, McKinlay SM, Brambilla D: The relative contributions of endocrine changes and social circumstances to depression in mid-aged women. J Health Soc Behav 28:345–363, 1987

McKinlay SM: The normal menopause transition: an overview. Maturitas 23:137–145, 1996

Morley JE: Androgens and aging. Maturitas 38:61–71, 2001

Morrison MF: Androgens in the elderly: will androgen replacement therapy improve mood, cognition, and quality of life in aging men and women? Psychopharmacol Bull 33:293–296, 1997

Nickelsen T, Lufkin EG, Riggs BL, et al: Raloxifene hydrochloride, a selective estrogen receptor modulator: safety assessment of effects on cognitive function and mood in postmenopausal women. Psychoneuroendocrinology 24:115–128, 1999

North American Menopause Society: Menopause Core Curriculum Study Guide. Cleveland, OH, North American Menopause Society, 2000, p 23

Notelovitz M: The clinical practice impact of the Women's Health Initiative: political vs biologic correctness. Maturitas 44:3–9, 2003

Paganini-Hill A, Henderson VW: The effects of hormone replacement therapy, lipoprotein cholesterol levels, and other factors on a clock drawing task in older women. J Am Geriatr Soc 44:818–822, 1996

Porter M, Penney GC, Russell D, et al: A population based survey of women's experience of the menopause. Br J Obstet Gynaecol 103:1025–1028, 1996

Ramachandran C, Fleisher D: Transdermal delivery of drugs for the treatment of bone diseases. Adv Drug Deliv Rev 42:197–223, 2000

Rapp SR, Espeland MA, Shumaker SA, et al: Effect of estrogen plus progestin on global cognitive function in postmenopausal women: the Women's Health Initiative Memory Study: a randomized controlled trial. JAMA 289:2663–2672, 2003

Resnick SM, Metter EJ, Zonderman AB: Estrogen replacement therapy and longitudinal decline in visual memory: a possible protective effect? Neurology 49:1491–1497, 1997

Rossouw JE, Anderson GL, Prentice RL, et al: Risks and benefits of estrogen plus progestin in healthy postmenopausal women: principal results from the Women's Health Initiative randomized controlled trial. JAMA 288:321–333, 2002

Rubinow DR, Schmidt PJ: Androgens, brain, and behavior. Am J Psychiatry 153:974–984, 1996

Saletu B, Brandstatter N, Metka M, et al: Double-blind, placebo-controlled, hormonal, syndromal and EEG mapping studies with transdermal oestradiol therapy in menopausal depression. Psychopharmacology (Berl) 122:321–329, 1995

Schmidt PJ, Roca CA, Bloch M, et al: The perimenopause and affective disorders. Semin Reprod Endocrinol 15:91–100, 1997

Schmidt PJ, Nieman L, Danaceau MA, et al: Estrogen replacement in perimenopause-related depression: a preliminary report. Am J Obstet Gynecol 183:414–420, 2000

Schneider LS, Small GW, Hamilton SH, et al: Estrogen replacement and response to fluoxetine in a multicenter geriatric depression trial. Fluoxetine Collaborative Study Group. Am J Geriatr Psychiatry 5:97–106, 1997

Scott RT Jr, Ross B, Anderson C, et al: Pharmacokinetics of percutaneous estradiol: a crossover study using a gel and a transdermal system in comparison with oral micronized estradiol. Obstet Gynecol 77:758–764, 1991

Seshadri S, Zornberg GL, Derby LE, et al: Postmenopausal estrogen replacement therapy and the risk of Alzheimer disease. Arch Neurol 58:435–440, 2001

Sherwin BB: Can estrogen keep you smart? Evidence from clinical studies. J Psychiatry Neurosci 24:315–321, 1999

Sherwin BB, Gelfand MM: Sex steroids and affect in the surgical menopause: a double-blind, cross-over study. Psychoneuroendocrinology 10:325–335, 1985

Shifren JL, Schiff I: The aging ovary. J Womens Health Gend Based Med (suppl 1)9:S3–S7, 2000

Shifren JL, Braunstein GD, Simon JA, et al: Transdermal testosterone treatment in women with impaired sexual function after oophorectomy. N Engl J Med 343:682–688, 2000

Shumaker SA, Legault C, Rapp SR, et al: Estrogen plus progestin and the incidence of dementia and mild cognitive impairment in postmenopausal women: the Women's Health Initiative Memory Study: a randomized controlled trial. JAMA 289:2651–2662, 2003

Silva I, Mor G, Naftolin F: Estrogen and the aging brain. Maturitas 38:95–100, 2001

Smith RN, Studd JW, Zamblera D, et al: A randomised comparison over 8 months of 100 micrograms and 200 micrograms twice weekly doses of transdermal oestradiol in the treatment of severe premenstrual syndrome. Br J Obstet Gynaecol 102:475–484, 1995

Smith YR, Giordani B, Lajiness-O'Neill R, et al: Long-term estrogen replacement is associated with improved nonverbal memory and attentional measures in postmenopausal women. Fertil Steril 76:1101–1107, 2001

Soares CN: Sex, hormones and depression: the impact of sex steroids on mood across the reproductive life cycle. Paper presented at the annual meeting of the American Psychiatric Association, San Francisco, CA, May 2003

Soares CN, Cohen LS: The perimenopause and mood disturbance. CNS Spectr 6:167–174, 2001

Soares CN, Almeida OP, Joffe H, et al: Efficacy of estradiol for the treatment of depressive disorders in perimenopausal women: a double-blind, randomized, placebo-controlled trial. Arch Gen Psychiatry 58:529–534, 2001a

Soares CN, Cohen LS, Otto MW, et al: Characteristics of women with premenstrual dysphoric disorder (PMDD) who did or did not report history of depression: a preliminary report from the Harvard Study of Moods and Cycles. J Womens Health Gend Based Med 10:873–878, 2001b

Soares CN, Poitras JR, Prouty J, et al: Efficacy of citalopram as a monotherapy or as an adjunctive treatment to estrogen therapy for perimenopausal and postmenopausal women with depression and vasomotor symptoms. J Clin Psychiatry 64:473–479, 2003

Stahl SM: Sex and psychopharmacology: is natural estrogen a psychotropic drug in women? Arch Gen Psychiatry 58:537–538, 2001

Steiner M: Female-specific mood disorders. Clin Obstet Gynecol 35:599–611, 1992

Stewart DE, Boydell KM: Psychologic distress during menopause: associations across the reproductive life cycle. Int J Psychiatry Med 23:157–162, 1993

Stone AB, Pearlstein TB: Evaluation and treatment of changes in mood, sleep, and sexual functioning associated with menopause. Obstet Gynecol Clin North Am 21:391–403, 1994

Strickler RC, Borth R, Cecutti A, et al: The role of oestrogen replacement in the climacteric syndrome. Psychol Med 7:631–639, 1977

Strickler R, Stovall DW, Merritt D, et al: Raloxifene and estrogen effects on quality of life in healthy postmenopausal women: a placebo-controlled randomized trial. Obstet Gynecol 96:359–365, 2000

Sumner BE, Grant KE, Rosie R, et al: Effects of tamoxifen on serotonin transporter and 5-hydroxytryptamine(2A) receptor binding sites and mRNA levels in the brain of ovariectomized rats with or without acute estradiol replacement. Brain Res Mol Brain Res 73:119–128, 1999

Szklo M, Cerhan J, Diez-Roux AV, et al: Estrogen replacement therapy and cognitive functioning in the Atherosclerosis Risk in Communities (ARIC) Study. Am J Epidemiol 144:1048–1057, 1996

Thompson J, Oswald I: Effect of oestrogen on the sleep, mood, and anxiety of menopausal women. Br Med J 2:1317–1319, 1977

Thompson DS, Spanier CA, Vogel VG: The relationship between tamoxifen, estrogen, and depressive symptoms. Breast J 5:375–382, 1999

U.S. Food and Drug Administration (FDA): FDA Talk Paper: FDA plans to evaluate results of Women's Health Initiative study for estrogen-alone therapy. March 2, 2004. Available at: http://www.fda.gov/bbs/topics/answers/2004/ans01281.html. Accessed March 4, 2004.

Westhoff C, Wieland D, Tiezzi L: Depression in users of depo-medroxyprogesterone acetate. Contraception 51:351–354, 1995

Wickelgren I: Estrogen stakes claim to cognition. Science 276:675–678, 1997

Wieland S, Belluzzi J, Hawkinson JE, et al: Anxiolytic and anticonvulsant activity of a synthetic neuroactive steroid Co 3-0593. Psychopharmacology (Berl) 134:46–54, 1997

Wihlback AC, Sundstrom-Poromaa I, Allard P, et al: Influence of postmenopausal hormone replacement therapy on platelet serotonin uptake site and serotonin 2A receptor binding. Obstet Gynecol 98:450–457, 2001

Wise PM, Krajnak KM, Kashon ML: Menopause: the aging of multiple pacemakers. Science 273:67–70, 1996

Wissink S, van der Burg B, Katzenellenbogen BS, et al: Synergistic activation of the serotonin-1A receptor by nuclear factor-kappa B and estrogen. Mol Endocrinol 15:543–552, 2001

Wolf OT, Kirschbaum C: Actions of dehydroepiandrosterone and its sulfate in the central nervous system: effects on cognition and emotion in animals and humans. Brain Res Brain Res Rev 30:264–288, 1999

Wolkowitz OM, Reus VI, Roberts E, et al: Dehydroepiandrosterone (DHEA) treatment of depression. Biol Psychiatry 41:311–318, 1997

Woolley CS: Effects of estrogen in the CNS. Curr Opin Neurobiol 9:349–354, 1999

Wyatt K, Dimmock P, Jones P, et al: Efficacy of progesterone and progestogens in management of premenstrual syndrome: systematic review. BMJ 323:776–780, 2001

Yaffe K, Ettinger B, Pressman A, et al: Neuropsychiatric function and dehydroepiandrosterone sulfate in elderly women: a prospective study. Biol Psychiatry 43:694–700, 1998a

Yaffe K, Grady D, Pressman A, et al: Serum estrogen levels, cognitive performance, and risk of cognitive decline in older community women. J Am Geriatr Soc 46:816–821, 1998b

Yaffe K, Krueger K, Sarkar S, et al: Cognitive function in postmenopausal women treated with raloxifene. N Engl J Med 344:1207–1213, 2001

Zumoff BV, Bradlow HL: Sex difference in the metabolism of dehydroisoandrosterone sulfate. J Clin Endocrinol Metab 51:334–336, 1980

Chapter 4

Mood Disorders, Midlife, and Reproductive Aging

Jamie A. Luff, M.D.

Khursheed Khine, M.D.

Peter J. Schmidt, M.D.

David R. Rubinow, M.D.

𝓘n this chapter, we focus on the potential relationship between the onset of affective disorders in women and the reproductive events of midlife and the perimenopause. First, we present background information relevant to the controversy surrounding the putative relationship between reproductive aging and mood disorders, review the endocrinology of this phase of a woman's life, and describe those methodologic problems that have hindered efforts to clarify the existence and nature of a potential relationship between the onset of depression and the perimenopause. Several emerging methodologic issues that may help resolve otherwise discrepant findings between previous observational studies and more recent randomized controlled trials are also emphasized. Second, we describe studies examining the prevalence, presentation, and pathophysiology of mood disorders occurring during the perimenopause and midlife. Finally, we discuss the clinical evaluation and management of these conditions.

Historical Perspectives

The nineteenth-century medical literature contained numerous case reports describing the onset of mood and behavioral disorders in women during midlife and reproductive aging. These early observations, in turn, led to speculations about the role of ovarian steroids in brain function and psychiatric illness, speculations supported by the anecdotal reports of the psychotropic actions of ovarian extracts. Nonetheless, in the psychiatric literature a debate ensued regarding the nature of these mood and behavioral disturbances and their connection to reproductive aging.

Descriptions of involutional-related syndromes in the nineteenth century ranged from minor depressive illnesses (like neurasthenia) to more severe forms of depressive illness with psychotic features. For example, Conklin (1889) described a syndrome reminiscent of minor depression or a mixed anxiety-depressive state occurring in the context of vasomotor symptoms and numerous somatic symptoms, whereas Maudsley (1867) reported a syndrome more akin to endogenous depression, in association with delusions of guilt and episodes of psychomotor agitation. The controversy surrounding these conditions was not about whether a menopausal mood syndrome existed but about how it should be classified.

The depression described by Maudsley in England was also described in Germany by Kraepelin in 1896 as a form of involutional melancholia (Kraepelin 1909). Although Kraepelin's description of involutional melancholia was not confined to women, his clinical presentation resembled Maudsley's climacteric melancholia: a particularly rigid and obsessive personality, no previous history of depression prior to the involutional period, no episodes of mania (distinguishing them from manic-depressive patients), a cross-sectional presentation with an agitated depression and hypochondriacal or nihilistic delusions, and a variable outcome. Both Kraepelin and Maudsley excluded involutional melancholia from manic-depressive psychosis and considered it a separate entity with a variable prognosis. Thus, on the basis of the Kraepelinian criterion of longitudinal outcome, this condition was neither manic-depressive psychosis (good outcome and eventual recovery) nor dementia praecox (poor outcome with deterioration). Similarly, Bleuler's description of schizophrenia (Bleuler 1924), with his emphasis on cross-sectional "symptomatology" rather than outcome, supported involutional melancholia as an independent diagnostic entity. The separateness of this syndrome was postulated on the basis of different symptomatology, different age at onset of index episode, different premorbid personality, and different family history. Subsequently, Stenstedt (1959) further distinguished menopause-related involutional patients from others with involutional depression by observing the former group to exhibit less severe symptoms and lower risk of affective disorder in family members.

Despite the debate over classification, a mood disorder called *involutional psychotic reaction* appeared in the first *Diagnostic and Statistical Manual: Mental Disorders* (DSM-I; American Psychiatric Association 1952). Indeed, following the successful isolation and synthesis of ovarian steroids and the subsequent widespread use of estrogen replacement therapy in the 1940s, investigators reported the therapeutic benefits of estrogen replacement in women with involutional melancholia. Thus, mainstream psychiatry accepted the existence of a type of mood disorder related to reproductive aging (albeit not without dissent; see Rosenthal 1968) and, in fact, inferred a causal association between the two events, given both the timing of onset and preliminary suggestions of the beneficial effects of estrogen replacement.

Prior to the third edition of the *Diagnostic and Statistical Manual of Mental Disorders* (DSM-III; American Psychiatric Association 1980), several investigators performed more systematic examinations of mood disorders occurring in association with midlife and reproductive aging. These studies were unable to confirm the existence of involutional melancholia, nor were they able to identify epidemiologic evidence for an increased prevalence of major depressive disorder during menopause. Thus, the earlier debate over the appropriate classification of involutional melancholia changed to skepticism about its existence as a distinct condition. Consequently, this classification was removed from DSM-IV and its text revision, DSM-IV-TR (American Psychiatric Association 1994, 2000). Moreover, these findings suggested that hormonal events did not underlie mood disorders occurring during midlife and reproductive aging.

In summary, several studies (Myers et al. 1984; Weissman 1979; Winokur 1973; Winokur and Cadoret 1975) provided evidence against the validity of the involutional melancholia construct, in that 1) there appeared to be no distinct symptom pattern; 2) there was no distinct pattern of previous episodes of depression in patients with menopause-related major depressive episodes; 3) there was no increased risk of suicide or psychiatric hospitalization during menopause; and 4) there appeared to be no increased prevalence of depression during menopause. Additionally, despite a generally higher prevalence rate of depression in females compared with males, some studies (Myers et al. 1984) reported a slightly lower 6-month prevalence rate of depression during the presumed menopausal or climacteric years than in younger age groups.

This evidence, however, is far from conclusive in refuting the existence of a menopause-related mood syndrome. See also Chapter 3, Effects of Reproductive Hormones and Selective Estrogen Receptor Modulators on the Central Nervous System During Menopause. Despite similar or lower point prevalence rates and similar clinical presentations of depression during menopause and at other times of life, one cannot infer that these syndromes share identical etiologies. Both Stenstedt (1959) and Brown et al. (1984) reported involutional-onset depression to be associated with a lower family history of depression than that observed in patients with early-onset depression. Further, in the study by Weissman (1979), 47% of the menopausal and 65% of the postmenopausal depressed women (as defined by age criteria) had no previous history of depression. Although the prevalence of histories of primary depression is not significantly in excess of that seen in the younger age group (44%), the substantially greater period of risk of developing an episode of depression in menopause or postmenopause group suggests that the percentage of primary depression is disproportionately high. Thus, although menopausal major depressions do not appear phenomenologically distinct, evidence suggests that they may differ from earlier onset depressions with respect to family history and age of index depressive episode. Further, epidemiologic and even phenomenological similarity does not entail causal identity. It is not unusual in medicine for phenomenologically similar disorders to have different precipitants or causes; for example, meningitis in both the neonate and the infant may present with fever, vomiting, and drowsiness, yet different pathogenic organisms are typically involved with each age group.

The presupposition that menopause-related affective syndromes, if they exist, are melancholic depressions is an additional confound that may have interfered with the identification and characterization of other affective syndromes (e.g., atypical depression) occurring at this time. In fact, many of the original reports described a clinical picture during menopause that was more consistent with a neurasthenia or minor depression. This suggestion is supported by several studies examining the prevalence of affective symptoms in menopausal women.

Winokur (1973) studied a sample of 71 consecutive female patients with an admission diagnosis of affective disorder and identified 28 patients as menopausal on the basis of at least a 3-year history of amenorrhea preceding admission. Winokur compared the risk of hospitalization for a depressive episode during the 3 years postmenopause of these 28 patients with the overall risk of developing an affective syndrome between ages 20 and 80 in the total sample of 71 women (i.e., the total number of depressive episodes divided by the number of years at risk). Because there was no significant difference between the risk of depression during the 3 years postmenopause and during the entire period of risk (ages 20–80 years), Winokur concluded the following: that menopause is not an important precipitant of episodes of affective disorder, that affective disorders are not more likely to occur during menopause; and that the study of menopause-associated depression is unlikely to promote further understanding of affective disorders. Winokur observed that the symptoms of depression and anxiety were so common during menopause, however, that an additional criterion for depression was imposed for these (but not the younger) subjects—that is, hospitalization—thus spuriously decreasing the rate of observed affective disorders during the 3 menopausal years. Given Winokur's observation of the high frequency of reports of menopause-related affective symptomatology in this group, it seems unwarranted to then conclude that there is "little value in looking specifically at the menopausal state for clues to the etiology of ordinary affective disorder" (Winokur 1973, p. 93).

Reproductive Events Related to Midlife, Perimenopause, and Postmenopause

Menopause has been defined as the permanent cessation of menstruation resulting from loss of ovarian activity. It is characterized endocrinologically by tonically elevated gonadotropin secretion (follicle-stimulating hormone [FSH], luteinizing hormone), persistently low levels of ovarian steroids (estradiol, progesterone), and relatively low (50% decrease, compared with younger age groups) androgen secretion (Couzinet et al. 2001). *Perimenopause* has been defined as the transitional period from reproductive to nonreproductive life (Santoro et al. 1996). As the perimenopause progresses, ovarian follicular depletion occurs, the ovary becomes less sensitive to gonadotropin stimulation, and a state of relative hypoestrogenism occurs; gonadotropin secretion is elevated across the menstrual cycle; ovulatory cycles are fewer; and menstrual cycle irregularity ensues. See also Chapter 2, Physiology and Symptoms of Menopause, and Chapter 7, Gynecologic Aspects of Perimenopause and Menopause. However, in contrast to postmenopause, episodic (not tonic) gonadotropin secretion is present, and both ovulation and normal premenopausal (or at times increased) estradiol secretion may occur (Burger et al. 1995; Santoro et al. 1996). Late perimenopause is characterized endocrinologically by persistent elevations of plasma FSH, sustained menstrual cycle irregularity with periods of amenorrhea, and hypoestrogenism. The levels of several other hormones that may also affect mood and behavior decrease with aging concomitant with changes in reproductive function. These hormones include androgens (testosterone and androstenedione; Burger et al. 1995; Couzinet et al. 2001), which begin to decline in the 20s and reach peak decline during the late 40s and 50s; dehydroepiandrosterone (DHEA); and insulin-like growth factors and binding proteins.

Not only is there evidence suggesting the importance of distinguishing between peri- and postmenopausal women with respect to treatment response characteristics (as discussed later), but studies have identified that the perimenopause has distinct endocrine characteristics, with early perimenopause (e.g., high gonadotropin levels and increased estradiol secretion) differing from late perimenopause (e.g., high gonadotropin levels and decreased estradiol secretion). Thus investigators have attempted to develop criteria to define the phases of reproductive aging more carefully and, therefore, facilitate the collection of more homogeneous samples to more precisely understand the interaction among the stage of ovarian decline, aging, and a variety of physiological end points. For example, the Stages of Reproductive Aging Workshop (STRAW) criteria for reproductive, perimenopausal (menopausal transition), and postmenopausal years developed by Soules et al. (2001) define the early perimenopause to include women with menstrual cycle irregularity (defined as a variable cycle length that differs from normal by more than 7 days) and elevated plasma FSH secretion. During late perimenopause, there is a continued elevation of FSH in conjunction with two or more skipped cycles and a period of amenorrhea lasting at least 60 days. This could include up to 1 year of amenorrhea, at which time the woman has entered early postmenopause.

Methodologic Problems in Investigations of the Relationship Among Mood Disturbance, Midlife, and Reproductive Aging

Methodologic problems in previous studies, related to the manner in which reproductive status and mood syndromes were defined, have compromised our ability to understand the role of reproductive aging in mood disorders and the role of estradiol in treating these disorders. See also Chapter 3, Effects of Reproductive Hormones and Selective Estrogen Receptor Modulators on the Central Nervous System During Menopause.

Characterizing Reproductive Status

Several criteria have been employed to define the reproductive status of women participating in studies of the relationship between menopause and mood. First, an age window of 45–55 years has been used to select perimenopausal subjects. Although the average age of menopause is 51 years, there is considerable individual variation in the age at onset of menopause, ranging from the early 40s to the late 50s. Adopting an age window as the sole selection criterion will inevitably result in the selection of a heterogeneous sample of women: some premenopausal, some perimenopausal, and some postmenopausal. Second, investigators have employed age combined with retrospective or prospective self-reports of menstrual cycle disturbance and have defined *menopause* as 6 months to 1 year of amenorrhea and *perimenopause* as menstrual cycle irregularity. However, self-reports of menstrual cycle irregularity cannot be used to reliably define reproductive status. Treloar (1981) observed that menstrual cycle irregularity is not confined to perimenopause and may occur frequently during other periods of reproductive life. Moreover, Kaufert et al. (1987) observed that among a sample of middle-aged women with menstrual cycle irregularity, as many women returned to normal menstrual cycle function as entered menopause (defined by 6 months of amenorrhea) during a 3-year period of follow-up. Finally, there is a 5%–10% probability that a woman will have menstrual bleeding even after 12 months of amenorrhea (Guthrie et al. 2002). The third criterion commonly used to define reproductive status has been the presence of elevated plasma gonadotropin (i.e., FSH) levels in the context of low plasma estradiol levels. However, perimenopause-related elevations in gonadotropins may be reversible, and in our sample of 310 women who had four serial FSH levels drawn every 2 weeks for 6 weeks, an elevated FSH (>20 IU/L) during the first sampling was not subsequently confirmed in 10% of cases (K. Khine, unpublished data, July 2003). A combination of age, menstrual cycle history, and plasma gonadotropin levels may be the most reliable method for selecting and characterizing the reproductive status of perimenopausal women, but it will not predict future reproductive function in every woman.

Defining Mood Syndromes

Another methodologic problem has been the failure to define midlife mood disorder as a syndrome (a condition meeting standardized diagnostic criteria) rather than an unintegrated set of symptoms. Mood symptoms differ from mood syndromes in their instruments of detection, their duration, and their impact. Structured interviews are employed in research settings to diagnose syndromes like depression, and these schedules introduce additional criteria to those present in DSM-IV-TR to ensure diagnostic homogeneity within samples and comparability across studies. For example, in addition to the presence of the DSM-IV core symptom criteria, the Structured Clinical Interview for DSM-IV (SCID; First et al. 1997) specifies that symptoms of depression must be present nearly every day for most of the day. The SCID also requires that the severity of depression be rated from mild to severe based on the number of symptoms in excess of those required for the diagnosis of minor or major depression and the level of functional impairment. In general, a structured diagnostic interview is the most reliable method for assessing the presence of a mood syndrome. In contrast, the cross-sectional scales employed in many studies measure the severity of depressive-like symptoms but do not assess either the longitudinal persistence of a core group of depressive symptoms or the level of functional impairment, both of which are important constituents of a depressive syndrome. Additionally, cross-sectional rating scales, such as the Center for Epidemiologic Studies Depression Scale, have restricted sampling intervals of 1–2 weeks and have reported sensitivity rates of only 75% (Roberts and Vernon 1983).

In addition to the importance of employing standardized psychiatric diagnostic interviews for establishing the presence of current and past psychiatric mood syndromes, investigators need to define and identify the type of mood syndromes that they are investigating. For example, both major and minor depressions exist, yet many studies focus only on the presence of major depression, with the exclusion of minor depression justified on the basis of its significance. Major depression has an estimated lifetime prevalence of 17%, and it affects approximately twice as many women as men (Kessler et al. 1994). The exact prevalence of minor depression is controversial because of differences in the diagnostic criteria used across studies; however, its prevalence is thought to approximate that of major depression (Johnson et al. 1992; Kessler et al. 1997). Minor depressions, by definition, have fewer and less severe symptoms than major depressions (Judd et al. 1994). Nonetheless, they are associated with disability comparable to that of major depression (Broadhead et al. 1990; Judd et al. 2002; Lopez and Murray 1998). Major depressions of moderate severity are not distinguished from minor depressions by family history (Angst 1997; Kendler and Gardner 1998), course (i.e., both major and minor depressions occur in subjects over their lifetimes; Judd et al. 1994), or biological characteristics (Akiskal et al. 1997; Kumar et al. 1998).

Mood Disturbances Occurring During Midlife and Reproductive Aging

Depressive Symptoms

Although postmenopause has not been associated with an increased risk of developing depression in women (Avis et al. 1994; Kaufert et al. 1992; McKinlay et al. 1987), depressive symptoms have been observed more frequently in perimenopausal women compared with postmenopausal women in some longitudinal, community-based studies (Hunter 1992; Matthews 1992).

Similarly, depressive-like symptoms have been evaluated in perimenopausal women attending gynecology clinics (Dennerstein et al. 1993; Hay et al. 1994; Stewart et al. 1992), with one study observing that up to 45% of the sample had high scores (consistent with clinically significant depression) on standardized rating scales for depression (Hay et al. 1994). In two additional studies, perimenopausal women reported significantly more symptoms than postmenopausal women (Dennerstein et al. 1993; Stewart et al. 1992). Thus, both clinic-based surveys and epidemiologic studies suggest the relevance of perimenopause in disturbances of mood in a substantial number of women.

Depressive Syndromes

Community-based surveys of the prevalence of affective *syndromes* (conditions meeting standardized diagnostic criteria, such as major or minor depression) have observed patterns of morbidity consistent with those reported in the surveys examining mood *symptoms*. Several epidemiologic studies examining gender- and age-related differences in the 6-month to 1-year prevalence of major depression reported no increased prevalence of major depression in women at midlife (age range: approximately 45–55 years; Kessler et al. 1993; Weissman et al. 1988). In contrast, a multinational study by Weissman and colleagues identified an increased hazard rate for the onset of depression in the cohort of women (but not men) between 45 and 50 years of age. The Study of Women's Health Across the Nation (SWAN; Bromberger et al. 2001) used a measure of "psychological distress" as a proxy for the syndrome of depression by requiring that core depressive symptoms (sadness, anxiety, and irritability) persist for at least 2 weeks. Similar to the studies of depressive symptoms, SWAN's initial cross-sectional survey observed that perimenopausal women reported significantly more "psychological distress" than either pre- or postmenopausal women (defined by self-reported menstrual cycle status; Bromberger et al. 2001). Moreover, the increased psychological distress appeared independent of the presence of vasomotor symptoms. These data, therefore, provide additional evidence supporting the role of perimenopause, but not postmenopause, in the development of mood disorders. On unipolar depression, see also Chapter 3, Effects of Reproductive Hormones and Selective Estrogen Receptor Modulators on the Central Nervous System During Menopause. On bipolar disorder, see also Chapter 5, Psychotic Illness in Women at Perimenopause and Menopause.

Anxiety Syndromes

There also is evidence that anxiety disorders, although less common than depressive disorders, are experienced by a considerable number of perimenopausal women (Hay et al. 1994) and that the frequency of episodes may increase during perimenopause (Ellen Freeman, M.D., unpublished communication, March 2004). New-onset panic disorder in perimenopause has been observed anecdotally and may be responsive to estrogen therapy; however, in our experience the frequent comorbidity of perimenopausal panic disorder and hot flashes and their shared symptomatology prevent one from readily separating the two phenomena. Thus, estradiol treatment may be effective for panic attacks; however, it is unclear if this improvement is secondary to relief of hot flashes (which may trigger as well as mimic panic attacks) or the result of the direct effects of estradiol on panic disorder. Moreover, both hot flashes and panic improve after treatment with selective serotonin reuptake inhibitors (SSRIs), suggesting a potential shared pathophysiology as well as treatment response characteristics.

Summary

Epidemiologic studies examining the prevalence of both affective symptoms and syndromes have documented that the majority of postmenopausal women do not experience a major depression associated with this phase of life. Nevertheless, several community-based and clinic-based surveys suggest that perimenopause is relevant to the development of affective disorders (Bromberger et al. 2001; Hay et al. 1994; Stewart et al. 1992) and that a substantial number of perimenopausal women do, in fact, experience a clinically significant affective syndrome.

Emerging Concepts

Recent studies of the relationship between reproductive aging and mood disturbance have used more reliable methods, both for establishing the presence or absence of mood syndromes (e.g., structured diagnostic interview) and for characterizing reproductive status (e.g., the STRAW criteria; Soules et al. 2001). These studies also have generated considerable debate, reflecting in part efforts to reconcile substantial differences in the results of observational studies compared with those from randomized controlled trials (RCTs) of hormone replacement therapy (HT). Thus, several new methodologic issues have been identified that may predict a differential response to changes in hormones (either endogenous or exogenous), including the phase of reproductive aging (i.e., late perimenopause or early menopause versus 5 years past last menses), the presence of menopausal symptoms, the duration of hypogonadism prior to receiving HT, and genetic polymorphisms that underlie differences in steroid responsivity. A differential response to estradiol in depression was reported by Appleby (1981), with perimenopausal but not postmenopausal women responding to estrogen therapy under randomized, placebo-controlled conditions (observations confirmed by several RCTs that have used standardized psychiatric diagnostic interviews to establish the presence of depression: Morrison et al. 2004; Schmidt et al. 2000; Soares et al. 2001). Similarly, a literature review and meta-analysis by Yaffe et al. (1998) concluded that the benefits of HT for cognitive function were limited to perimenopausal women compared with postmenopausal women and suggested that the beneficial effects of HT were secondary to the concurrent improvement in menopausal symptoms. A subsequent meta-analysis of a similar literature performed by LeBlanc (2001) confirmed Yaffe's suggestion and observed that the presence of symptoms (e.g., hot flashes, sleep disturbance, or mood disturbance) predicted a beneficial effect of HT on cognition. Similarly, studies in both animals and humans suggest that a short duration of hypogonadism prior to initiation of estrogen therapy is associated with beneficial effects on both measures of cognition (Gibbs 2000; Resnick and Henderson 2002; Zandi et al. 2002) and atherosclerotic plaque formation (Brownley et al. 2004; Mikkola and Clarkson 2002). These findings are consistent with the observed differences in treatment response between perimenopausal or recently menopausal and older postmenopausal women (the former more likely to be symptomatic) (Dennerstein et al. 1993; Stewart et al. 1992). In addition, these findings introduce the concept of the critical window for the efficacy of HT. For example, nonhuman primate studies have shown that initiation of HT is associated with cardioprotection when administered immediately after oophorectomy but not after 30 months (approximately 6 human years; Mikkola and Clarkson 2002). This critical-window construct has been proposed as an explanation for some of the discrepant findings between the observational studies (many of which included younger, more symptomatic women) and the RCTs related to the Women's Health Initiative (Shumaker et al. 2003; Writing Group for the Women's Health Initiative Investigators 2002), which principally included older asymptomatic women (Grodstein et al. 2003; Resnick and Henderson 2002). Finally, independent of stage of reproductive life or duration of hypogonadism, several studies that used both plasma lipid levels and cognitive outcome measures suggest that the effects of sex steroids may be influenced by the presence of polymorphisms in specific steroid receptors (Herrington et al. 2002; Yaffe et al. 2002).

The evidence that younger perimenopausal but not older postmenopausal women respond to estrogen therapy suggests that those mood disorders occurring in perimenopausal women are caused by *changes* in hormones (e.g., withdrawal or fluctuations) rather than by prolonged sex steroid deficiency. The possibility that the change in or acute withdrawal from ovarian steroids is the relevant factor in the pathophysiology of these conditions suggests several mechanisms that may be involved in the onset of mood disorders during the perimenopause. First, because perimenopause may be associated with prolonged and increased estradiol secretion, it is possible that these increased levels of estradiol compromise central nervous system function (Hung et al. 2003). Alternatively, mood disorders may occur secondary to estrogen withdrawal in a manner similar to that proposed for opiate withdrawal syndromes.

Neuroregulatory Potential of Alterations in Ovarian Estradiol Secretion

Results from animal studies demonstrate that gonadal steroids influence several of the neuroregulatory systems thought to be involved in both the pathophysiology of affective disorders and the efficacy of antidepressant therapies (McEwen et al. 1997; Rachman et al. 1998; Woolley and Schwartz-kroin 1998). In some, but not all (Rubinow et al. 1998), experimental paradigms, estradiol, like antidepressants, has been observed to inhibit serotonin reuptake transporter mRNA (Pecins-Thompson et al. 1998) and decrease activity (downregulation and uncoupling from its G-protein) at 5-hydroxy-tryptamine 1A (5-HT$_{1A}$) receptors (Clarke and Maayani 1990; Thomas et al. 1997). In addition to classic neurotransmitter systems, several neural signaling systems have been identified as potential mediators of the therapeutic actions of antidepressants and electroconvulsive therapy (ECT), including CREB (cyclic AMP response element–binding) protein and BDNF (brain-derived neurotrophic factor) (Nestler et al. 1989), based on observations that these systems are modulated by a range of therapies effective in depression (e.g., serotonergic agents, noradrenergic agents, and ECT) and exhibit a pattern of change consistent with the latency to therapeutic efficacy for most antidepressants (Duman et al. 1997). For example, antidepressants increase the expression and activity of CREB in certain brain regions (e.g., hippocampus) (Nibuya et al. 1996) and regulate (in a brain region–specific manner) activity of genes with a cAMP response element (Duman et al. 1997). Genes for BDNF and its receptor trkB have been proposed as potential targets for antidepressant-related changes in CREB activity (Duman et al. 1997). Similarly, estradiol has been reported to influence many of these same neuroregulatory processes. Specifically, ovariectomy has been reported to decrease, and estradiol to increase, BDNF levels in the forebrain and hippo-campus (Sohrabji et al. 1994b). Estrogen also increases CREB activity (Zhou et al. 1996) and trkA (Sohrabji et al. 1994a) in the rat brain. In contrast, an estradiol-induced decrease in BDNF has been reported to mediate estradiol's regulation of dendritic spine formation in hippocampal neurons (Murphy et al. 1998). Thus, the therapeutic potential of gonadal steroids in depression is suggested not only by their widespread actions on neurotransmitter systems but also by certain neuroregulatory actions shared by both estrogen and traditional therapies for depression (i.e., antidepressants, ECT).

Possible Causes of Depression During Midlife and Reproductive Aging

Hormone Withdrawal or Deficiency Theory

Plasma Hormone Studies

Several reports indirectly support a role for abnormalities of reproductive hormones during the perimenopause in depression: 1) Hormone replacement beneficially affects both hot flashes and mood in hypogonadal women (Brincat et al. 1984; Ditkoff et al. 1991; Sherwin et al. 1985; Steingold et al. 1985), and 2) lower gonadotropin levels are sometimes observed in post-menopausal depressed women compared with asymptomatic comparison groups (Altman et al. 1975; Amsterdam et al. 1983; Brambilla et al. 1990; Guicheney et al. 1988). Perimenopausal women with depressive symptoms have been reported to have lower plasma estrone levels (Ballinger 1990) than nondepressed perimenopausal women, and an association has been de-scribed between increased plasma FSH levels and depression (Huerta et al. 1995). In contrast, three studies of perimenopausal and postmenopausal women observed either no diagnosis-related differences in plasma estradiol and FSH (Saletu et al. 1996) or no correlation between plasma levels of es-trogens or androgens and the severity of depressive symptoms (Barrett-Con-nor et al. 1999; Cawood and Bancroft 1996).

In a study of 21 women with their first episode of depression occurring during perimenopause and 21 asymptomatic perimenopausal control sub-jects (Schmidt et al. 2002), we were unable to confirm previous reports of lower basal plasma levels of luteinizing hormone (Altman et al. 1975; Am-sterdam et al. 1983; Brambilla et al. 1990; Guicheney et al. 1988) or estrone (Ballinger 1990) in perimenopausal and postmenopausal women with de-pression. In additional, no diagnosis-related differences in basal plasma lev-els of FSH, estradiol, testosterone, or free testosterone were observed. These data are consistent with those of Barrett-Connor et al. (1999) and of Cawood and Bancroft (1996), who, as described above, found no correlation between mood symptoms and plasma levels of estrone, estradiol, or testosterone.

The limitations of basal hormonal measures notwithstanding, these data suggest that depressed perimenopausal women cannot be distinguished from nondepressed perimenopausal women on the basis of abnormal ovarian hormone secretion.

In addition to ovarian hormones, age-related differences in the function of several other physiologic systems have been observed in both animals and humans. Some of these differences may occur coincident with perimenopause and, therefore, may potentially contribute to mood dysregulation at this time. Although postmenopausal women have been reported to exhibit increased stress-induced plasma norepinephrine levels as compared with premenopausal women (Matthews 1992), only one previous study (Ballinger 1990) reported elevated urinary cortisol levels in perimenopausal women reporting depressive symptoms as compared with asymptomatic control subjects. No systematic study has been performed of hypothalamic-pituitary-adrenal axis function in untreated perimenopausal depressed women.

A role for the adrenal androgen DHEA and its sulfated metabolite (DHEA-S) in the regulation of mood state also has been suggested by both its effects on neural physiology (Baulieu and Robel 1998; Majewska et al. 1990) and its potential synthesis within the central nervous system (Zwain and Yen 1999). Moreover, in clinical trials, DHEA administration has been reported to improve mood in some (Bloch et al. 1999; Morales et al. 1994; Wolkowitz et al. 1999), but not all, studies (Wolf et al. 1997). The potential role of DHEA in the onset of depression may be particularly relevant at midlife given the declining levels of DHEA production that occur with aging and the accelerated decrease in DHEA levels reported in women, but not men, during midlife (Laughlin and Barrett-Connor 2000). It is possible, therefore, that declining secretion (or abnormally low secretion) of DHEA may interact with perimenopause-related changes in ovarian function to trigger the onset of depression in some women. We (Schmidt et al. 2002) measured morning plasma levels of DHEA, DHEA-S, and cortisol in a sample of women with the first onset of depression during perimenopause and in nondepressed women matched for age and reproductive status. Depressed perimenopausal women had significantly lower levels of both plasma DHEA and DHEA-S, but not cortisol, as compared with control subjects (Schmidt et al. 2002). These findings are consistent with several previous studies suggesting an association between DHEA levels and mood. First, plasma DHEA levels correlated with the severity of depressive symptoms in a group of postmenopausal women, with lower levels of DHEA associated with higher depression scores (Barrett-Connor et al. 1999). In two other studies, a positive correlation between plasma DHEA-S levels and feelings of well-being was observed in groups of peri- and postmenopausal women (Cawood and Ban-croft 1996). The observation that DHEA secretion, but not adrenal glucocor-ticoid secretion, differed in depressed and nondepressed women suggests that depression during perimenopause may differ from that occurring at other periods in life.

Perimenopausal depressions may not be distinguished from major de-pressive disorder on the basis of phenomenology, course, or family or per-sonal history of mood disorder. Nonetheless, the relevance of changes in pituitary-ovarian function to depression during perimenopause is suggested by two findings: First, in some perimenopausal depressed women, mood symptoms improve concurrently with the restoration of ovarian function (Daly et al. 2003). Second, estradiol therapy may have mood-enhancing ef-fects in perimenopausal women with depression.

Trials of Hormone Therapy

Controlled studies that used synthetic forms of estrogen in the treatment of depression have yielded mixed results. Estrogen has been reported to im-prove mood (albeit inconsistently: Campbell 1976; Coope 1981; George et al. 1973) in the following samples: 1) perimenopausal and postmenopausal women reporting depressive symptoms (Montgomery et al. 1987; Saletu et al. 1995; Sherwin 1988), 2) postmenopausal women with depression un-responsive to traditional antidepressant therapy (Klaiber et al. 1979), and 3) nondepressed menopausal women not experiencing hot flashes (Ditkoff et al. 1991).

We (Schmidt et al. 2000) examined the therapeutic efficacy of estradiol replacement in 34 women (approximately half of whom had no prior history of depression) with perimenopausal depression under double-blind, pla-cebo-controlled conditions. After 3 weeks of estradiol, depression rating scale scores were significantly decreased compared to baseline scores and significantly lower than scores for the women receiving placebo. A full or partial therapeutic response was seen in 80% of subjects on estradiol and in 22% of those on placebo, consistent with the observed effect size (0.69) in a meta-analysis of studies examining estrogen's effects on mood (Zweifel and O'Brien 1997). The therapeutic response to estrogen was observed in both major and minor depression as well as in women with and without hot flashes. These data suggest that estrogen's effect on depression is not solely a product of its ability to reduce the distress of hot flashes.

These findings are consistent with data from Montgomery et al. (1987) and Saletu et al. (1995) suggesting the beneficial effects of estrogen on mood in perimenopausal women reporting depressive symptoms. Two more recent studies, by Soares et al. (2001) and Morrison et al. (2004), extended these observations. First, Soares and colleagues (2001) reported a significant and beneficial effect of estrogen replacement compared with placebo in women with perimenopause-related major depression (as defined by the PRIME MD [Primary Care Evaluation of Mental Disorders] study [Spitzer et al. 1995]), and they also reported that baseline plasma estradiol levels did not predict response to estrogen treatment. Second, Morrison and colleagues (2004) observed that estrogen was no more effective than placebo in postmenopausal depressed women, in contrast to previous results in perimenopausal women. These data emphasize that the stage of reproductive aging may predict response to estrogen, as originally reported by Appleby et al. (1981). Thus, perimenopausal women who are undergoing changes in reproductive function may be more responsive to estrogen than postmenopausal women, whose hormonal changes have long since stabilized.

As noted earlier, a relationship between DHEA and depression has been suggested by reports of alterations in plasma DHEA levels in depression (both decreased and increased) and initial reports of antidepressant-like effects of DHEA (either as monotherapy or combined with traditional antidepressant agents). We examined under double-blind placebo-controlled conditions the therapeutic efficacy of DHEA as monotherapy in men ($n=23$) and women ($n=23$) ages 45–65 years with midlife-onset depression. A significant improvement in depression severity was observed in both men and women on DHEA compared with both baseline and placebo conditions. The response to DHEA did not differ in men and women for any outcome measure. These data suggest, therefore, the potential of declining DHEA secretion alone or in combination with altered ovarian function in the onset of mood disorders during midlife in some men and women.

Hot Flashes and Dysphoria—The Domino Theory

A wealth of epidemiologic evidence demonstrates the co-occurrence of both hot flashes and depression in women during perimenopause (Hunter 1992; Jaszmann et al. 1969; Joffe et al. 2002; Matthews 1992; McKinlay et al. 1987). In a randomized controlled trial of 16 hypogonadal (peri- and postmenopausal) women, Schiff et al. (1979) showed that hot flashes, sleep, and mood all improved after treatment with conjugated estrogens. Based on these findings, it has been suggested that hot flashes and perimenopausal depression share the same pathophysiology or that there is a linear, causal relationship between them (i.e., hot flashes lead to sleep disturbances, which in turn lead to dysphoria). However, epidemiologic evidence also suggests that hot flashes and depression can also occur independently and are mutually dissociable phenomena (Avis et al. 2001; Bromberger et al. 2001). In addition, as mentioned earlier, there are women with perimenopausal depression without hot flashes whose depression responds to estrogen treatment (Schmidt et al. 2000). Further, as shown by Soares et al. (2001), in women successfully treated for depression and hot flashes, estradiol withdrawal results in a return of hot flashes, but *not* necessarily depression. Thus, while the two frequently coexist, hot flashes are neither necessary nor sufficient to cause depression. See Chapter 3, Effects of Reproductive Hormones and Selective Estrogen Receptor Modulators on the Central Nervous System During Menopause.

Life Events, Social Support, and Aging

Some but not all studies have suggested that both midlife and perimenopause are characterized by stressful life events and that perimenopausal depression may occur secondary to an increased number of stressful events, including personal losses (Cooke and Greene 1981). These stressors include the following: 1) alterations in family roles, 2) changing social support networks, 3) interpersonal losses, and 4) the physical effects of aging. However, a causal role for such environmental factors has not been demonstrated. Midlife, and in particular the perimenopause, is not uniformly characterized by stressful life changes such as children leaving the home, becoming a grandparent, loss of employment, divorce or widowhood, or the onset of medical illness (Dennerstein et al. 2001). Although these may be common events, they are not universal experiences, nor are they necessarily specific to the midlife. Furthermore, women's reactions to such life events are not uniform. There are certainly positive corollaries to the empty nest syndrome as well. A woman may instead experience the pleasures of being a grandmother or enjoy the freedoms she is afforded after her children have left home or following retirement from a demanding job (Ballinger et al. 1979; Dennerstein et al. 2002). Therefore, these life events alone cannot explain the increased vulnerability to depression that some women are subject to during this time.

We (Schmidt et al. 2004) found that women who developed depression during the perimenopause did not report more major losses (such as divorce, death in the family, or job loss) or "empty nest" events (children or other loved ones leaving the home) than matched control subjects. Thus perimenopausal depressions do not appear to be simply secondary to an increase in personal losses or the empty nest syndrome. These depressed women did report more negative events (e.g., related to work, school, relationships, or finances) than control subjects and also appeared to demonstrate an increased vulnerability to the negative impact of these events.

Several factors such as genetic predisposition (Caspi et al. 2003; Kendler et al. 1995), self-efficacy (Maciejewski et al. 2001), overall health, and social support (Seeman and Crimmins 2001) may differentially modify the negative impact of life events and may determine whether negative events trigger the onset of depression. It is possible, therefore, that these variables may mediate the effects of negative life events on mood in susceptible perimenopausal women, resulting in depression. (However, it is important to note that a woman's depressed state at the time of interview may color her perception of both the quantity and the impact of negative events in her recent past.)

It appears then that models describing menopause as a life crisis may misrepresent the negative impact of this developmental state or at least the universality of such an impact (McKinlay et al. 1987). The determinants of an individual's response to stressors, whether associated with the midlife or other developmental stages, are likely multifactorial and complex. It remains unclear which factors determine personal response to crisis, whether it is positive, resulting in goal achievement, mastery, and a feeling of satisfaction with one's self and one's contributions (Dennerstein et al. 2001), or negative, resulting in symptoms of emotional distress, low self-esteem, and depression (Erikson 1966).

Summary

Perimenopausal depression is not simply the effect of abnormalities in ovarian steroid production, nor is it merely secondary to severe hot flashes or personal losses. Nonetheless, data suggest that each of these factors may play a role in perimenopausal depression and could potentially cause depression in certain women; however, many of these same factors also are present in the majority of perimenopausal women who do not develop depression. Thus the mediating or protective factors involved in the development of depression at this time remain to be determined.

Management

From both research and clinical perspectives, the assessment of perimenopause-related depression should include a careful history focused on the following: 1) the prominence of the affective and behavioral symptoms relative to somatic symptoms such as hot flashes or vaginal dryness; 2) the presence of any past history of depression or hypomania, to compare the similarity of current symptoms with those of previous episodes; 3) possible comorbid or preexisting conditions; 4) the temporal relationship between the severity of mood symptoms and possible changes in menstrual cycle function (regular to irregular); 5) the frequency of estrogen-sensitive somatic symptoms, such as hot flashes, which may predict the effectiveness of estrogen therapy in treating mood and behavioral symptoms; 6) the current social and vocational context; 7) other symptoms that may affect self-esteem and that may be responsive to estrogen therapy, such as sexual dysfunction (caused by urogenital changes); and 8) the presence of contraindications to estrogen therapy, such as a personal or family history of breast cancer. The differential diagnosis of perimenopause-related depression includes the following: dysphoria secondary to hot flash–induced dyssomnia; depression secondary to adverse or stressful life events; recurrent depression; and medical illness (e.g., hypothyroidism) presenting as depression. Reproductive status may be characterized by serial plasma FSH or estradiol levels to confirm the presence of perimenopause and to track improvements in mood if they occur in relation to changes in pituitary-ovarian hormone secretion.

The decision to prescribe estradiol for perimenopausal depression must further be informed by associated risks and the availability of alternative treatments (such as DHEA, phytoestrogen, or testosterone supplementation). The Women's Health Initiative Study demonstrated that continuous administration of one form of estrogen (conjugated estrogens) in comnination with one form of progesterone (medroxyprogesterone acetate) is associated with an increased risk of dementia, heart attacks, stroke, blood clots, and breast cancer, particularly when administered many years after menopause (Rapp et al. 2003; Shumaker et al. 2003; Wassertheil-Smoller et al. 2003; Writing Group for the Women's Health Initiative Investigators 2002). Thus the potential risks for cardiovascular morbidity and breast cancer after prolonged estrogen therapy appear to offset the benefits of estrogen therapy as a first-line treatment for depression. In addition, several adequate treatments for depression exist, and therefore the first-line medication for perimenopausal women with depression is a traditional antidepressant such as an SSRI. Indeed, the reports of therapeutic benefits of SSRIs in hot flashes support a more prominent role for these medications in the management of perimenopausal depression. Nonetheless, treatment of depression with estradiol could be considered as follows: 1) as a treatment alternative for the approximately 50% of ambulatory depressed patients who do not respond to a conventional, first-line intervention (Fava et al. 1996); 2) for women who refuse to take psychotropic agents or who otherwise prefer treatment with estradiol; and 3) for women who will be undertaking treatment with estradiol for other acute symptoms (e.g., hot flashes) and who therefore could delay treatment with antidepressants until determining whether estradiol treatment was sufficient. Although estradiol treatment is no longer considered appropriate for prophylaxis, it still is reasonably prescribed for acute symptoms and syndromes, including depression.

In addition to the possible antidepressant efficacy of estrogen in perimenopausal depression, some, but not all (Amsterdam et al. 1999), studies
have suggested that response to some antidepressants (i.e., SSRIs) may be
enhanced by the use of estrogen therapy in perimenopausal (Soares et al.,
personal communication, September 2003) and postmenopausal women
(Schneider et al. 1997, 2001). Consequently, if not otherwise contraindicated, estrogen augmentation may be of value in the treatment of perimenopausal depressed women who are antidepressant nonresponders. Finally,
progestin may induce a dysphoric state in some women receiving estrogen
therapy; however, progestin-induced dysphorias are not uniformly experienced in all women, nor are predictors of the dysphoric response known.
Thus, progestins should not be contraindicated in the presence of an antidepressant response to estradiol in a depressed perimenopausal woman (and
are advised in women with a uterus).

Alternative hormonal treatment strategies include DHEA (available over
the counter), phytoestrogens, SERMs, and testosterone supplementation.
The potential roles in perimenopausal depression for phytoestrogens and
SERMs remain to be investigated (see Chapter 3, Effects of Reproductive
Hormones and Selective Estrogen Receptor Modulators on the Central Nervous System During Menopause, and Chapter 7, Gynecologic Aspects of
Perimenopause and Menopause), whereas DHEA may have an antidepressant effect in some women; however, the results of trials evaluating DHEA's
efficacy as a monotherapy in depression are pending. Reports of testosterone's effects on libido suggest the use of this strategy to augment libido in
some women (at midlife or during perimenopause) with decreased libido
despite treatment with either SSRIs or estradiol therapy. As a caveat, the
safety of long-term androgen administration in this age group has not been
fully established, and women risk the development of hirsutism, acne, and
oily skin, as well as the more serious potential effects of initiating or stimulating hormone-sensitive malignancies. As is true for other types of depression, psychotherapy is an important adjunct to pharmacological or hormonal
interventions, and it can prove crucial in women for whom menopause holds
negative meaning (e.g., a hysterectomy can be a traumatic loss for some
women) and in those who have significant life stressors and poor social supports.

Conclusion

The relationship between the onset of depressive illness and reproductive
aging has been a source of controversy. Epidemiologic and clinic-based studies that have distinguished between the perimenopause (a time of consider-

able variability in ovarian hormone secretion) and postmenopause (a time when hormonal changes have long since stabilized) have suggested that in some middle-aged women, the perimenopause is associated with an increased vulnerability to depression. Additional support for this suggestion is provided by double-blind, randomized controlled trials documenting the therapeutic efficacy of estradiol in perimenopausal depressed women but not in postmenopausal depressed women. Our future efforts should abandon the all-or-none controversy and should be directed toward understanding the determinants and consequences of the variability that we see in the following: 1) the response to change in reproductive endocrine function; 2) the response, whether therapeutic or adverse, to hormone therapy; 3) the impact of duration of hypogonadism; and 4) the behavioral effects of the large array of hormone receptor agonists and modulators.

References

Akiskal HS, Judd LL, Gillin C, et al: Subthreshold depressions: clinical and polysomnographic validation of dysthymic, residual and masked forms. J Affect Disord 45:53–63, 1997

Altman N, Sachar EJ, Gruen PH, et al: Reduced plasma LH concentration in postmenopausal depressed women. Psychosom Med 37:274–276, 1975

American Psychiatric Association: Diagnostic and Statistical Manual: Mental Disorders. Washington, DC, American Psychiatric Association, 1952

American Psychiatric Association: Diagnostic and Statistical Manual of Mental Disorders, 3rd Edition. Washington, DC, American Psychiatric Association, 1980

American Psychiatric Association: Diagnostic and Statistical Manual of Mental Disorders, 4th Edition. Washington, DC, American Psychiatric Association, 1994

American Psychiatric Association: Diagnostic and Statistical Manual of Mental Disorders, 4th Edition, Text Revision. Washington, DC, American Psychiatric Association, 2000

Amsterdam J, Garcia-Espana F, Fawcett J, et al: Fluoxetine efficacy in menopausal women with and without estrogen replacement. J Affect Disord 55:11–17, 1999

Amsterdam JD, Winokur A, Lucki I, et al: Neuroendocrine regulation in depressed postmenopausal women and healthy subjects. Acta Psychiatr Scand 67:43–49, 1983

Angst J: Minor and recurrent brief depression, in Dysthymia and the Spectrum of Chronic Depressions. Edited by Akiskal HS, Cassano GB. New York, Guilford, 1997, pp 183–190

Appleby L, Montgomery J, Studd J: Oestrogens and affective disorders, in Progress in Obstetrics and Gynaecology. Edited by Studd J. Edinburgh, Churchill Livingstone, 1981, pp 289–302

Avis NE, Brambilla D, McKinlay SM, et al: A longitudinal analysis of the association between menopause and depression: results from the Massachusetts Women's Health Study. Ann Epidemiol 4:214–220, 1994

Avis NE, Stellato R, Crawford S, et al: Is there a menopausal syndrome? Menopausal status and symptoms across racial/ethnic groups. Soc Sci Med 52:345–356, 2001

Ballinger S: Stress as a factor in lowered estrogen-levels in the early postmenopause. Ann N Y Acad Sci 592:95–113, 1990

Ballinger S, Cobbin D, Krivanek J, et al: Life stresses and depression in the menopause. Maturitas 1:191–199, 1979

Barrett-Connor E, von Muhlen D, Laughlin GA, et al: Endogenous levels of dehydroepiandrosterone sulfate, but not other sex hormones, are associated with depressed mood in older women: the Rancho Bernardo Study. J Am Geriatr Soc 47:685–691, 1999

Baulieu E-E, Robel P: Dehydroepiandrosterone (DHEA) and dehydroepiandrosterone sulfate (DHEAS) as neuroactive neurosteroids. Proc Natl Acad Sci U S A 95:4089–4091, 1998

Bleuler E: Textbook of Psychiatry. New York, Macmillan, 1924

Bloch M, Schmidt PJ, Danaceau MA, et al: Dehydroepiandrosterone treatment of mid-life dysthymia. Biol Psychiatry 45:1533–1541, 1999

Brambilla F, Maggioni M, Ferrari E, et al: Tonic and dynamic gonadotropin secretion in depressive and normothymic phases of affective disorders. Psychiatry Res 32:229–239, 1990

Brincat M, Studd JWW, O'Dowd T, et al: Subcutaneous hormone implants for the control of climacteric symptoms: a prospective study. Lancet 1:16–18, 1984

Broadhead WE, Blazer DG, George LK, et al: Depression, disability days, and days lost from work in a prospective epidemiologic survey. JAMA 264:2524–2528, 1990

Bromberger JT, Meyer PM, Kravitz HM, et al: Psychologic distress and natural menopause: a multiethnic community study. Am J Public Health 91:1435–1442, 2001

Brown RP, Sweeney J, Loutsch E, et al: Involutional melancholia revisited. Am J Psychiatry 141:24–28, 1984

Brownley KA, Hinderliter AL, West SG, et al: Cardiovascular effects of 6 months of hormone replacement therapy versus placebo: differences associated with years since menopause. Am J Obstet Gynecol 190:1052–1058, 2004

Burger HG, Dudley EC, Hopper JL, et al: The endocrinology of the menopausal transition: a cross-sectional study of a population-based sample. J Clin Endocrinol Metab 80:3537–3545, 1995

Campbell S: Double-blind psychometric studies on the effects of natural estrogens on post-menopausal women, in The Management of the Menopause and Post-Menopausal Years. Edited by Campbell S. Lancaster, England, MTP Press Ltd, 1976, pp 149–158

Caspi A, Sugden K, Moffitt TE, et al: Influence of life stress on depression: moderation by a polymorphism in the 5-HTT gene. Science 301:291–293, 2003

Cawood EHH, Bancroft J: Steroid hormones, the menopause, sexuality and well-being of women. Psychol Med 26:925–936, 1996

Clarke WP, Maayani S: Estrogen effects on 5-HT$_{1A}$ receptors in hippocampal membranes from ovariectomized rats: functional and binding studies. Brain Res 518:287–291, 1990

Conklin WJ: Some neuroses of the menopause. Transactions of the American Association of Obstetrics and Gynecology 2:301–311, 1889

Cooke DJ, Greene JG: Types of life events in relation to symptoms at the climacterium. J Psychosom Res 25:5–11, 1981

Coope J: Is oestrogen therapy effective in the treatment of menopausal depression? J R Coll Gen Pract 31:134–140, 1981

Couzinet B, Meduri G, Lecce MG, et al: The postmenopausal ovary is not a major androgen-producing gland. J Clin Endocrinol Metab 86:5060–5066, 2001

Daly RC, Danaceau MA, Rubinow DR, et al: Concordant restoration of ovarian function and mood in perimenopausal depression. Am J Psychiatry 160:1842–1846, 2003

Dennerstein L, Smith AMA, Morse C, et al: Menopausal symptoms in Australian women. Med J Aust 159:232–236, 1993

Dennerstein L, Lehert P, Dudley E, et al: Factors contributing to positive mood during the menopausal transition. J Nerv Ment Dis 189:84–89, 2001

Dennerstein L, Dudley E, Guthrie J: Empty nest or revolving door? A prospective study of women's quality of life in midlife during the phase of children leaving and re-entering the home. Psychol Med 32:545–550, 2002

Ditkoff EC, Crary WG, Cristo M, et al: Estrogen improves psychological function in asymptomatic postmenopausal women. Obstet Gynecol 78:991–995, 1991

Duman RS, Heninger GR, Nestler EJ: A molecular and cellular theory of depression. Arch Gen Psychiatry 54:597–606, 1997

Erikson EH: Eight ages of man. Int J Psychiatry 2:281–307, 1966

Fava M, Abraham M, Alpert J, et al: Gender differences in Axis I comorbidity among depressed outpatients. J Affect Disord 38:129–133, 1996

First MB, Spitzer RL, Williams JB, et al: Structured Clinical Interview for DSM-IV Axis I Disorders (SCID-I), clinician version. Washington, DC, American Psychiatric Association, 1997

George GCW, Utian WH, Beaumont PJV, et al: Effect of exogenous oestrogens on minor psychiatric symptoms in postmenopausal women. S Afr Med J 47:2387–2388, 1973

Gibbs RB: Long-term treatment with estrogen and progesterone enhances acquisition of a spatial memory task by ovariectomized aged rats. Neurobiol Aging 21:107–116, 2000

Grodstein F, Clarkson TB, Manson JE: Understanding the divergent data on postmenopausal hormone therapy. N Engl J Med 348:645–650, 2003

Guicheney P, Léger D, Barrat J, et al: Platelet serotonin content and plasma tryptophan in peri- and postmenopausal women: variations with plasma oestrogen levels and depressive symptoms. Eur J Clin Invest 18:297–304, 1988

Guthrie J, Dennerstein L, Burger H: How reliably does 12-month amenorrhea define final menstrual period? Data from a longitudinal study (letter). Climacteric 5:92, 2002

Hay AG, Bancroft J, Johnstone EC: Affective symptoms in women attending a meno-
    pause clinic. Br J Psychiatry 164:513–516, 1994

Herrington DM, Howard TD, Hawkins GA, et al: Estrogen-receptor polymorphisms
    and effects of estrogen replacement on high-density lipoprotein cholesterol in
    women with coronary disease. N Engl J Med 346:967–974, 2002

Huerta R, Mena A, Malacara JM, et al: Symptoms at perimenopausal period: its asso-
    ciation with attitudes toward sexuality, life-style, family function, and FSH lev-
    els. Psychoneuroendocrinology 20:135–148, 1995

Hung AJ, Stanbury MG, Shanabrough M, et al: Estrogen, synaptic plasticity and hy-
    pothalamic reproductive aging. Exp Gerontol 38:53–59, 2003

Hunter M: The South-East England longitudinal study of the climacteric and post-
    menopause. Maturitas 14:117–126, 1992

Jaszmann L, van Lith ND, Zaat JCA: The perimenopausal symptoms: the statistical
    analysis of a survey: part A. Med Gynaecol Sociol 4:268–277, 1969

Joffe H, Hall JE, Soares CN, et al: Vasomotor symptoms are associated with depres-
    sion in perimenopausal women seeking primary care. Menopause 9:392–398,
    2002

Johnson J, Weissman MM, Klerman GL: Service utilization and social morbidity as-
    sociated with depressive symptoms in the community. JAMA 267:1478–1483,
    1992

Judd LL, Rapaport MH, Paulus MP, et al: Subsyndromal symptomatic depression: a
    new mood disorder? J Clin Psychiatry 55:18–28, 1994

Judd LL, Schettler PJ, Akiskal HS: The prevalence, clinical relevance, and public
    health significance of subthreshold depressions. Psychiatr Clin North Am
    25:685–698, 2002

Kaufert PA, Gilbert P, Tate R: Defining menopausal status: the impact of longitudinal
    data. Maturitas 9:217–226, 1987

Kaufert PA, Gilbert P, Tate R: The Manitoba Project: a re-examination of the link be-
    tween menopause and depression. Maturitas 14:143–155, 1992

Kendler KS, Gardner CO Jr: Boundaries of major depression: an evaluation of DSM-
    IV criteria. Am J Psychiatry 155:172–177, 1998

Kendler KS, Kessler RC, Walters EE, et al: Stressful life events, genetic liability, and
    onset of an episode of major depression in women. Am J Psychiatry 152:833–
    842, 1995

Kessler RC, McGonagle KA, Swartz M, et al: Sex and depression in the National Co-
    morbidity Survey, I: lifetime prevalence, chronicity and recurrence. J Affect Dis-
    ord 29:85–96, 1993

Kessler RC, McGonagle KA, Zhao S, et al: Lifetime and 12-month prevalence of DSM-
    III-R psychiatric disorders in the United States: results from the National Co-
    morbidity Survey. Arch Gen Psychiatry 51:8–19, 1994

Kessler RC, Zhao S, Blazer DG, et al: Prevalence, correlates, and course of minor de-
    pression and major depression in the National Comorbidity Survey. J Affect Dis-
    ord 45:19–30, 1997

Klaiber EL, Broverman DM, Vogel W, et al: Estrogen therapy for severe persistent de-
    pressions in women. Arch Gen Psychiatry 36:550–554, 1979

Kraepelin E: Psychiatrie: ein Lehrbuch für Studierende und Ärzte. Leipzig, Barth, 1909

Kumar A, Jin Z, Bilker W, et al: Late-onset minor and major depression: early evidence for common neuroanatomical substrates detected by using MRI. Proc Natl Acad Sci U S A 95:7654–7658, 1998

Laughlin GA, Barrett-Connor E: Sexual dimorphism in the influence of advanced aging on adrenal hormone levels: the Rancho Bernardo Study. J Clin Endocrinol Metab 85:3561–3568, 2000

LeBlanc ES, Janowsky J, Chan BKS, et al: Hormone replacement therapy and cognition: systematic review and meta-analysis. JAMA 285:1489–1499, 2001

Lopez AD, Murray CCJL: The global burden of disease, 1990–2020. Nat Med 4:1241–1243, 1998

Maciejewski PK, Prigerson HG, Mazure CM: Sex differences in event-related risk for major depression. Psychol Med 31:593–604, 2001

Majewska MD, Demirgören S, Spivak CE, et al: The neurosteroid dehydroepiandrosterone sulfate is an allosteric antagonist of the $GABA_A$ receptor. Brain Res 526:143–146, 1990

Matthews KA: Myths and realities of the menopause. Psychosom Med 54:1–9, 1992

Maudsley H: The physiology and pathology of the mind. New York, D Appleton, 1867

McEwen BS, Alves SE, Bulloch K, et al: Ovarian steroids and the brain: implications for cognition and aging. Neurology 48 (suppl 7):S8–S15, 1997

McKinlay JB, McKinlay SM, Brambilla D: The relative contributions of endocrine changes and social circumstances to depression in mid-aged women. J Health Soc Behav 28:345–363, 1987

Mikkola TS, Clarkson TB: Estrogen replacement therapy, atherosclerosis, and vascular function. Cardiovasc Res 53:605–619, 2002

Montgomery JC, Brincat M, Tapp A, et al: Effect of oestrogen and testosterone implants on psychological disorders in the climacteric. Lancet 1:297–299, 1987

Morales AJ, Nolan JJ, Nelson JC, et al: Effects of replacement dose of dehydroepiandrosterone in men and women of advancing age. J Clin Endocrinol Metab 78:1360–1367, 1994

Morrison MF, Kallan MJ, Ten Have T, et al: Lack of efficacy of estradiol for depression in postmenopausal women: a randomized, controlled trial. Biol Psychiatry 55:406–412, 2004

Murphy DD, Cole NB, Segal M: Brain-derived neurotrophic factor mediates estradiol-induced dendritic spine formation in hippocampal neurons. Proc Natl Acad Sci U S A 95:11412–11417, 1998

Myers JK, Weissman MM, Tischler GL, et al: Six-month prevalence of psychiatric disorders in three communities. Arch Gen Psychiatry 41:959–967, 1984

Nestler EJ, Terwilliger RZ, Duman RS: Chronic antidepressant administration alters the subcellular distribution of cyclic AMP–dependent protein kinase in rat frontal cortex. J Neurochem 53:1644–1647, 1989

Nibuya M, Nestler EJ, Duman RS: Chronic antidepressant administration increases the expression of cAMP response element-binding protein (CREB) in rat hippocampus. J Neurosci 16:2365–2372, 1996

Pecins-Thompson M, Brown NA, Bethea CL: Regulation of serotonin re-uptake transporter mRNA expression by ovarian steroids in rhesus macaques. Brain Res Mol Brain Res 53:120–129, 1998

Rachman IM, Unnerstall JR, Pfaff DW, et al: Estrogen alters behavior and forebrain c-*fos* expression in ovariectomized rats subjected to the forced swim test. Proc Natl Acad Sci U S A 95:13941–13946, 1998

Rapp SR, Espeland MA, Shumaker SA, et al: Effect of estrogen plus progestin on global cognitive function in postmenopausal women: the Women's Health Initiative Memory Study: a randomized controlled trial. JAMA 289:2663–2672, 2003

Resnick SM, Henderson VW: Hormone therapy and risk of Alzheimer disease: a critical time. JAMA 288:2170–2172, 2002

Roberts RE, Vernon SW: The Center for Epidemiologic Studies Depression Scale: its use in a community sample. Am J Psychiatry 140:41–46, 1983

Rosenthal S: The involutional depressive syndrome. Am J Psychiatry 124:21–35, 1968

Rubinow DR, Schmidt PJ, Roca CA: Estrogen-serotonin interactions: implications for affective regulation. Biol Psychiatry 44:839–850, 1998

Saletu B, Brandstatter N, Metka M, et al: Double-blind, placebo-controlled, hormonal, syndromal and EEG mapping studies with transdermal oestradiol therapy in menopausal depression. Psychopharmacology (Berl) 122:321–329, 1995

Saletu B, Brandstatter N, Metka M, et al: Hormonal, syndromal and EEG mapping studies in menopausal syndrome patients with and without depression as compared with controls. Maturitas 23:91–105, 1996

Santoro N, Brown JR, Adel T, et al: Characterization of reproductive hormonal dynamics in the perimenopause. J Clin Endocrinol Metab 81:1495–1501, 1996

Schiff I, Regestein Q, Tulchinsky D, et al: Effects of estrogens on sleep and psychological state of hypogonadal women. JAMA 242:2405–2407, 1979

Schmidt PJ, Nieman L, Danaceau MA, et al: Estrogen replacement in perimenopause-related depression: a preliminary report. Am J Obstet Gynecol 183:414–420, 2000

Schmidt PJ, Murphy JH, Haq N, et al: Basal plasma hormone levels in depressed perimenopausal women. Psychoneuroendocrinology 27:907–920, 2002

Schmidt PJ, Murphy JH, Haq NA, et al: Stressful life events, personal losses, and perimenopause-related depression. Arch Womens Ment Health 7:19–26, 2004

Schneider LS, Small GW, Hamilton SH, et al: Estrogen replacement and response to fluoxetine in a multicenter geriatric depression trial. Am J Geriatr Psychiatry 5:97–106, 1997

Schneider LS, Small GW, Clary CM: Estrogen replacement therapy and antidepressant response to sertraline in older depressed women. Am J Geriatr Psychiatry 9:393–399, 2001

Seeman TE, Crimmins E: Social environment effects on health and aging: integrating epidemiologic and demographic approaches and perspectives. Ann N Y Acad Sci 954:88–117, 2001

Sherwin BB: Affective changes with estrogen and androgen replacement therapy in surgically menopausal women. J Affect Disord 14:177–187, 1988

Sherwin BB, Gelfand MM: Differential symptom response to parenteral estrogen and/ or androgen administration in the surgical menopause. Am J Obstet Gynecol 151:153–160, 1985

Shumaker SA, Legault C, Rapp SR, et al: Estrogen plus progestin and the incidence of dementia and mild cognitive impairment in postmenopausal women: the Women's Health Initiative Memory Study: a randomized controlled trial. JAMA 289:2651–2662, 2003

Soares CN, Almeida OP, Joffe H, et al: Efficacy of estradiol for the treatment of depressive disorders in perimenopausal women: a double-blind, randomized, placebo-controlled trial. Arch Gen Psychiatry 58:529–534, 2001

Sohrabji F, Greene LA, Miranda RC, et al: Reciprocal regulation of estrogen and NGF receptors by their ligands in PC12 cells. J Neurobiol 25:974–988, 1994a

Sohrabji F, Miranda RC, Toran-Allerand CD: Estrogen differentially regulates estrogen and nerve growth factor receptor mRNAs in adult sensory neurons. J Neurosci 14:459–471, 1994b

Soules MR, Sherman S, Parrott E, et al: Executive summary: Stages of Reproductive Aging Workshop (STRAW). Fertil Steril 76:874–878, 2001

Spitzer RL, Kroenke K, Linzer M, et al: Health-related quality of life in primary care patients with mental disorders: results from the PRIME-MD 1000 Study. JAMA 274:1511–1517, 1995

Steingold KA, Laufer L, Chetkowski RJ, et al: Treatment of hot flashes with transdermal estradiol administration. J Clin Endocrinol Metab 61:627–632, 1985

Stenstedt A: Involutional melancholia: an etiologic, clinical and social study of endogenous depression in later life, with special reference to genetic factors. Acta Psychiatr Neurol Scand 34 (suppl 127):1–71, 1959

Stewart DE, Boydell K, Derzko C, et al: Psychologic distress during the menopausal years in women attending a menopause clinic. Int J Psychiatry Med 22:213–220, 1992

Thomas ML, Bland DA, Clarke CH, et al: Estrogen regulation of serotonin (5-HT) transporter and 5-HT$_{1A}$ receptor mRNA in female rat brain (abstract). Society for Neuroscience Abstracts 23:1501, 1997

Treloar AE: Menstrual cyclicity and the pre-menopause. Maturitas 3:249–264, 1981

Wassertheil-Smoller S, Hendrix SL, Limacher M, et al: Effect of estrogen plus progestin on stroke in postmenopausal women: the Women's Health Initiative: a randomized trial. JAMA 289:2673–2684, 2003

Weissman MM: The myth of involutional melancholia. JAMA 242:742–744, 1979

Weissman MM, Leaf PJ, Tischler GL, et al: Affective disorders in five United States communities. Psychol Med 18:141–153, 1988

Winokur G: Depression in the menopause. Am J Psychiatry 130:92–93, 1973

Winokur G, Cadoret R: The irrelevance of the menopause to depressive disease, in Topics in Psychoendocrinology. Edited by Sachar EJ. New York, Grune & Stratton, 1975, pp 59–66

Wolf OT, Neumann O, Hellhammer DH, et al: Effects of a two-week physiological dehydroepiandrosterone substitution on cognitive performance and well-being in healthy elderly women and men. J Clin Endocrinol Metab 82:2363–2367, 1997

Wolkowitz OM, Reus VI, Keebler A, et al: Double-blind treatment of major depression with dehydroepiandrosterone. Am J Psychiatry 156:646–649, 1999

Woolley CS, Schwartzkroin PA: Hormonal effects on the brain. Epilepsia 39 (suppl 8):S2–S8, 1998

Writing Group for the Women's Health Initiative Investigators: Risks and benefits of estrogen plus progestin in healthy postmenopausal women: principal results from the Women's Health Initiative randomized controlled trial. JAMA 288:321–333, 2002

Yaffe K, Sawaya G, Lieberburg I, et al: Estrogen therapy in postmenopausal women: effects on cognitive function and dementia. JAMA 279:688–695, 1998

Yaffe K, Lui LY, Grady D, et al: Estrogen receptor 1 polymorphisms and risk of cognitive impairment in older women. Biol Psychiatry 51:677–682, 2002

Zandi PP, Carlson MC, Plassman BL, et al: Hormone replacement therapy and incidence of Alzheimer disease in older women: the Cache County Study. JAMA 288:2123–2129, 2002

Zhou Y, Watters JJ, Dorsa DM: Estrogen rapidly induces the phosphorylation of the cAMP response element binding protein in rat brain. Endocrinology 137:2163–2166, 1996

Zwain IH, Yen SSC: Dehydroepiandrosterone: biosynthesis and metabolism in the brain. Endocrinology 140:880–887, 1999

Zweifel JE, O'Brien WH: A meta-analysis of the effect of hormone replacement therapy upon depressed mood. Psychoneuroendocrinology 22:189–212, 1997

Chapter 5

Psychotic Illness in Women at Perimenopause and Menopause

Jayashri Kulkarni,
M.B.B.S., M.P.M., Ph.D., F.R.A.N.Z.C.P.

$\mathcal{T}$ he role of sex steroids in brain function is receiving increasing research attention (see Chapter 3 in this volume), although the clinical consequences of estrogen loss for brain function are only now being scrutinized. In this chapter, I describe new findings on the role of estrogen in treating psychotic mental illnesses such as schizophrenia and bipolar affective disorder.

Women and Schizophrenia: A Midlife View

History

In former times, some clinicians, including Kraepelin (1909–1915) and Kretschmer (1921), believed that schizophrenia stemmed partly from a disturbed hormone balance. In 1921, Kretschmer wrote, "In schizophrenics, one has always, and with good reason, paid special attention to these organs [the sexual glands]....Firstly, there is the fact that schizophrenic disorders have a marked preference for puberty." Diczfalusy and Lauritzen (1961) reviewed past attempts to analyze estrogen levels in the blood and urine of women with schizophrenia.

Krafft-Ebing (1896) had noticed that some women became psychotic during the premenstrual or low-estradiol phase of the menstrual cycle. Kraepelin (1909–1915) suggested a separate diagnostic category, the "menstrual psychosis." Bleuler (1943) described a "loss of ovarian functioning," associated with late-onset schizophrenia in women. Seven studies (between 1933 and 1955) showed lower than usual levels of estrogens in women with schizophrenia, but sample sizes were small and laboratory techniques were crude. Baruk et al. (1950) examined vaginal smears to discover the influence of estrogen on mental states and found "hypoestrogenisms" in 23 cases of "dementia praecox." As Riecher-Rossler et al. (1997) pointed out, such early findings are of special interest because at the time, there was no neuroleptic therapy, so the findings cannot reflect a neuroleptic effect.

In 1943, Bleuler undertook an unsystematic clinical trial prescribing a "combined ovarian anterior pituitary hormone" to women with late-onset schizophrenia starting at age 40. Mall (1960) systematically examined estrogen fluctuations in 167 women with schizophrenia by measuring urine estrogen excretion over a 24-hour period and also examining vaginal cytology and taking basal temperatures. He concluded that there were two different forms of psychosis—a "hypofollicular" and a "hyperfollicular" one. Mall gave estrogens to women with the hypofollicular form, stating that "hypofollicular psychoses can be healed relatively easily with this substitution therapy" (p. 223). However, there are few details of the study in the account by Riecher-Rossler et al. (1997) of Mall's research.

It is unclear why these early clinicians' findings were forgotten, ignored, or not followed up. However, their observations led to the idea that hypoestrogenism might be linked to schizophrenia in women. According to an international consensus, the key gender differences observed in schizophrenia are that women develop it at a later age than men and that the incidence of schizophrenia in women increases after menopause.

To explain these differences, researchers such as Hafner (1987) and Seeman (1982) suggested that women are somehow "protected" against the early onset of schizophrenia and that estrogen may be the protective agent. Neither of these key researchers based the estrogen protection hypothesis on epidemiologic findings alone. Both used clinical data and animal studies to support their hypothesis.

More recently, epidemiologic, clinical, and neuroendocrine animal studies have been investigating the estrogen protection hypothesis, which is discussed in detail in the next sections.

More Recent Studies

Animal Studies

Initial animal studies exploring the effect of estradiol on dopamine receptors gave varied results, depending on the dose and duration of estradiol administered. Clopton and Gordon (1986) administered low doses of estrogen (10 µg/kg/day estradiol benzoate) to ovariectomized female Sprague-Dawley rats and found that administering low doses of estrogen decreased dopamine receptor sensitivity. Fields and Gordon (1982) demonstrated an apparent ability of estrogen to downregulate brain dopamine receptors and postulated that this might lead to some useful pharmacological treatment for tardive dyskinesia.

Neither of these studies investigated the dose effect or the length of time for which estrogen administration remained effective. Using more rigorous methods, Ferretti et al. (1992) studied the effects of high- and low-dose estradiol administration for both short and long periods (up to 120 days) in both male and female rats. The researchers concluded that low doses of estradiol diminished the density of dopamine D_2 receptors, particularly in young female rats, but that high doses of estradiol triggered complex responses that differed in males compared with females.

In a review of the effects of sex steroids on brain dopamine transmission, Di Paolo (1994) emphasized the biphasic impact of estrogen as a function of time and dose. Di Paolo theorized that the initial dopamine hyposensitivity response induced by estrogen may be a direct effect in which dopamine D_2 receptors couple to G-proteins. The second hyposensitive effect exerted by high-dose estradiol administration or because of a lengthier administration may be mediated via an estrogen-stimulated hormone such as prolactin. Another hypothesis put forward by Di Paolo (1994) is that chronic estradiol administration increases D_2 receptor density in the anterior pituitary by a genomic mechanism. Di Paolo's study (1994) revealed an increase in mRNA levels in the anterior pituitary but not in the striatum of rats given long-term estradiol.

More recently, Fink and colleagues (1999) found that estradiol selectively stimulates the expression of the 5-hydroxytryptamine 2A ($5-HT_{2A}$) receptor mRNA in the dorsal raphe nucleus of female rats. They also found that a single pulse of estradiol induced a significant increase in the density of $5-HT_{2A}$ receptors in the female rat forebrain. Fink et al. suggested that serotonergic (5-HT) mechanisms might be partly responsible for schizophrenia, particularly in view of the action of atypical antipsychotic drugs such as clozapine and risperidone. The estradiol effect on $5-HT_{2A}$ receptors may explain the "psychoprotectant" role of estrogen in schizophrenia. Although the precise mechanisms whereby estrogen affects dopamine and serotonin receptors remain unclear, it appears that estrogen may have some therapeutic role in treating schizophrenia.

Clinical Studies

Although men and women have the same overall incidence and lifetime prevalence of schizophrenia, the onset of symptoms occurs sooner in men (Hafner and an der Heiden 1997). Schizophrenia in women tends to be relatively mild at first, with increasing severity later on, whereas symptoms in men usually taper off with advancing years (Ciompi 1993). This disparity may be connected to the swifter decrease in serotonin and dopamine receptors with age in men (Wong et al. 1984). Reports suggest that women respond better than men to antipsychotic medication and that women of childbearing age respond better than older, postmenopausal women (Seeman 1995).

Some clinical case reports indicate that psychotic symptoms may occur cyclically in women with schizophrenia, peaking during the late luteal phase when estrogen levels are at their lowest. Women with schizophrenia often require lower doses of neuroleptics premenopausally than after menopause. Riecher-Rossler et al. (1997) tested the hypothesis that the symptoms of schizophrenia vary with menstrual cycle phase in 32 acutely admitted women who had histories of regular menstrual cycles. These women had more hospital admissions during the premenstrual (i.e., low-estrogen) phase than in their high-estrogen phase. This study also found a significant inverse relationship between estradiol levels and the severity of psychotic symptoms. Furthermore, all 32 patients had markedly low estradiol levels throughout their cycle.

Older women with schizophrenia have to cope with cognitive decline, long-term medication, and other treatments as well as the effect of serious disabilities and depleted estrogen levels. A large body of literature strongly supports the concept that late-onset schizophrenia—a predominantly female illness—is characterized by a particularly severe symptomatology and course (Riecher-Rossler et al. 1997).

Late-onset schizophrenia is unquestionably more common in women than in men—a finding that has been frequently replicated (Faraone et al. 1994). However, the late onset has not been definitely linked to estrogen withdrawal (Howard et al. 1994; Pearlson and Rabins 1988). Nonetheless, the striking correlation between waning estrogen levels in the fourth decade and the exacerbation of existing illness or the increasingly common presentation of schizophrenia in women of this age cannot be ignored. In support of the estrogen protection hypothesis is the observation that during pregnancy, when estrogen levels are very high, many women with severe schizophrenia have diminished symptoms. In addition, the onset of postpartum psychosis coincides with a sharp, fast drop in estrogen levels. Further support for a therapeutically protective effect of estrogen comes from our own work on the use of estrogen for treating women with schizophrenia.

We conducted an open-label pilot study in which 11 women of childbearing age with schizophrenia were given 0.02 mg oral ethinyl estradiol as an adjunct to antipsychotic drug treatment for 8 weeks, and we compared their progress with that of a similar group who received only antipsychotic drugs (Kulkarni et al. 1996). The group taking estrogen recovered rapidly from acute psychotic symptoms and also reported greater overall improvement in their general health status.

Subsequently, we conducted a dose-finding study to discover the optimal use of estradiol in women with schizophrenia (Kulkarni et al. 2001). This was a three-arm, double-blind, placebo-controlled, 28-day study on women with a diagnosis of DSM-IV (American Psychiatric Association 1994) schizophrenia in which 12 women received 50 μg transdermal estradiol plus a standardized antipsychotic drug, 12 women received 100 μg transdermal estradiol plus antipsychotic drug, and 12 women received placebo plus antipsychotic drug.

The main finding from this study was that the addition of 100 μg transdermal estradiol to the antipsychotic medication gave the best outcomes for women with schizophrenia, compared with a group that received 50 μg transdermal estradiol with antipsychotic drugs and a group that received only antipsychotic drugs. The clinical improvement in key psychotic symptoms was significantly greater in those given the adjunctive 100 μg estrogen.

Currently, we are conducting a double-blind, placebo-controlled trial of 100 μg transdermal estradiol in women of childbearing age with schizophrenia (Kulkarni et al. 2002). To date, we have enrolled 69 of a targeted 90 women in the study. Each subject was enrolled in the trial for 28 days, having received a baseline psychopathology and hormone assessment followed by weekly assessments. At each assessment, psychopathology was measured using the Positive and Negative Syndrome Scale (PANSS). Hormone assays were done for serum estrogen, progesterone, prolactin, luteinizing hormone (LH), follicle-stimulating hormone (FSH), and testosterone. A menstrual cycle interview was used to stage each patient's menstrual phase. A battery of cognitive tests was administered that included tests of the higher brain functions most likely to be affected by estrogen. This strategy targeted visuospatial and verbal memory skills, also serving as an evaluation of more general cognitive abilities. Patients were randomly assigned to an active-treatment group receiving 100 μg estradiol via a skin patch or an identical placebo patch group. All patients received antipsychotic drug treatment, which was administered according to a protocol using doses between 3 and 7 mg/day of risperidone, the dose depending on the patient's clinical state. Each patient's score from baseline, in total, positive, negative, and general PANSS scores, was calculated at each visit.

We found no statistically significant differences between the 37 women who received 100 µg adjunctive transdermal estradiol and the 32 women receiving adjunctive transdermal placebo in terms of age, menstrual cycle phase, diagnosis, or antipsychotic drug dose. The group receiving estrogen (100 µg) had a more significant decrease than the placebo group in psychotic symptoms as measured by the PANSS ($P<0.001$). Similar effects were observed for the positive, negative, and general PANSS subscales across time. The changes in hormonal data across 28 days for the two groups revealed that the estrogen group had significantly higher mean estrogen levels and lower LH levels. There were no significant differences in progesterone, FSH, prolactin, or testosterone levels between the estrogen-treated and placebo groups. Women receiving estrogen performed significantly better on working memory tests and tended ($P>0.01$) to perform better on the visual reproduction and verbal memory tasks.

Our interim results reinforce the evidence in favor of adding 100 µg of transdermal estradiol to achieve greater relief of psychotic symptoms in women with DSM-IV schizophrenia. As indicated by its effect on the pituitary measured by LH assay, administering 100 µg of transdermal estradiol provides unconjugated estrogen in a form and dose that positively affect central nervous system neurotransmitter systems. This finding agrees with the estrogen hypothesis formulated by Hafner (1987). At this writing, our study is nearing completion, and final results will be reported.

Menopause and Schizophrenia

Seeman reported that women of childbearing age tend to require lower neuroleptic or antipsychotic doses of medication than perimenopausal and postmenopausal women to recover from an acute episode of psychosis and that they attain remission faster. The doses of medication required to maintain recovery at the later stages of life increase as the "psychoprotective" effect of estrogen declines (Seeman 2002). In addition, longitudinal outcomes, which are better for women than for men for the first 15 years of illness (Angermeyer et al. 1990; Davidson and McGlashan 1997; Mason et al. 1995), gradually even out (Opjordsmoen 1991; Steinmeyer et al. 1989). Therefore, at or around menopause, women's relative advantage with respect to schizophrenia outcomes wanes or vanishes. Seeman (2002) reported a longitudinal chart review of 20 women admitted for schizophrenia treatment showing a postmenopausal decline in function, compared with that in their 40s, that she attributed to a drop in estrogen levels with advancing age. Married women did no better than others with regard to estrogen decline. The biggest difference detected was that the four patients who deteriorated most significantly each had a child they had previously given up for adoption. Seeman speculated that the advent of menopause for a woman whose only child had been adopted signaled an especially dramatic end to the possibility of childbearing. She concluded that among the various physical and psychosocial changes that occur at menopause, the symptoms of schizophrenia may be aggravated at that time as a direct or indirect result of estrogen withdrawal. She proposed that declining estrogen levels may have a significant effect via cognitive pathways, by activating or suppressing genes that are estrogen dependent or through a direct impact on the neurotransmitters that help to regulate higher cognitive functioning.

Studies by Jeste et al. (1995) revealed that women with late-onset schizophrenia were more likely to have paranoid delusions but better premorbid adjustment. The diagnosis of schizophrenia in elderly women can be difficult and can be complicated by accompanying medical conditions or the effect of multiple medications. In treating women with schizophrenia, particularly around menopause, the optimal use of estrogens and progestins is still to be authoritatively determined. However, in the near future, a greater variety of hormone therapies will be available, such as second and subsequent generations of the selective estrogen receptor modulators (SERMs)—for example, raloxifene—that specifically work on targeted organs. Knowledge about the precise impact of later-generation SERMs on cognition, mood, and psychiatric conditions awaits further research. In women who have perimenopausal psychotic relapses in a cyclical manner, cycle-modulated antipsychotic treatment or monophasic contraceptive pills have been proposed as a means of modulating serum levels of estrogen (Braendle et al. 2001).

As already stated, women face increased risks of relapse or a first psychotic episode at or near the menopause. The current debate about the use of estrogen treatment or hormone therapy (HT) has focused primarily on its use to alleviate troubling symptoms of perimenopause and to prevent various medical disorders. As women with schizophrenia approach menopause, existing medical conditions may be exacerbated because of lengthy treatment with antipsychotic drugs, especially those that reduce circulating estrogen levels through hyperprolactinemia. Hence, because schizophrenia is a serious, disabling, and frequently life-threatening illness, women with schizophrenia should be assessed carefully as they enter menopause. The use of HT for perimenopausal symptoms, as well as mental states, in these women should be considered in light of the medical arguments for and against use of HT. See Chapter 6, Medical Aspects of Perimenopause and Menopause.

To date, health professionals have sometimes been rather remiss in their history taking about menstrual irregularities, amenorrhea, galactorrhea, and symptoms of menopause (such as hot flashes, reduced libido, changes in vaginal lubrication, and anorgasmia), often to the woman's detriment. Preventive health screening such as Pap smears and mammograms may be forgotten. Smoking, a sedentary lifestyle, poor nutrition, and obesity may further complicate the health of women with schizophrenia, leading to diabetes mellitus, cardiovascular disease, and increased risk of cancer. Patients with schizophrenia accompanied by iatrogenic early menopause are open to potentially serious consequences such as osteoporosis. In cases of hyperprolactinemia with secondary estrogen deficiency, ongoing laboratory investigations are essential to evaluate the patient's hormonal state and decide whether to use atypical antipsychotic medications that produce little or no hyperprolactinemia. The addition of estrogen to the treatment regimen may be advised, bearing in mind the caveats in Chapter 6, Medical Aspects of Perimenopause and Menopause, and Chapter 7, Gynecologic Aspects of Perimenopause and Menopause.

Cognition in Women With Schizophrenia During Perimenopause and Menopause

Components of Cognition

Cognition is a general term that describes the totality of human information processing. It includes memory, higher intellectual functioning and psychomotor skills, problem solving, pattern recognition, learning, language processing, and abstract reasoning. Memory is a vital aspect of cognition and in itself has a number of component parts that are localized to different parts of the brain. It is now generally agreed that short-term memory and long-term memory are mediated by two separate systems (Baddeley and Warrington 1970; Milner 1972). Learning is concerned with encoding and storing information, and the forgetting of information often occurs because that material cannot be retrieved. The inability to retrieve previously learned material may occur because it had never been properly encoded (Tulving 1972) or because the recall or recognition cues are not effective. Either or both of these possibilities could impair long-term memory (Sherwin 2003). *Working memory* refers to the ability to "hold in mind" and manipulate information over a short period of time to make a response (Baddeley et al. 1986).

In patients with schizophrenia, in particular those in midlife or later life, the changes in working memory and long- and short-term memory are incapacitating in both social and work settings. Cognitive rehabilitation, also known as cognitive remediation, aims to remedy or correct deficits in cognitive functions such as memory, executive functioning, and concentration. This form of treatment is very different from cognitive-behavioral therapy, which tries to modify the actual content of thoughts and beliefs. Antipsychotic medications cannot completely or reliably reverse the cognitive disturbances in schizophrenia. Therefore, nonpharmacological interventions provide an additional treatment tool. Although women with schizophrenia often have widespread gaps in cognitive functioning, the deficits are highly variable and individual. For example, a patient may have memory lapses but retain or preserve such functions as sustained attention or executive abilities. The challenge in therapy is to focus on those deficits that have the most detrimental impact on a particular person. Many midlife women with schizophrenia describe serious problems arising from the loss of working memory that hamper their day-to-day lives. In the past, women rarely took up new careers or parenting in midlife, so cognitive rehabilitation as a vital part of their overall treatment was often overlooked. But today things are changing.

Wykes and co-workers (1999) compared what they termed *neurocognitive rehabilitation* with a form of intensive occupational therapy. They described modules for improving cognitive flexibility, working memory, and planning. Such therapy may be very effective in improving the quality of life for older women with schizophrenia. Special attention is usually given to the rehabilitation of young people with early psychotic illness, because these patients clearly need intensive intervention to ensure a good outcome. However, older women and those midway through their lives who experience a first episode of psychosis, or who relapse as a result of biological changes such as hormonal fluctuations or some social precipitating factor, deserve equally intensive care to regain a quality of life lost through the illness.

Community Intervention and Support for Women at Perimenopause and Menopause With Psychotic Illness

The process of deinstitutionalization was inaugurated in the 1960s when seriously ill psychiatric patients were discharged into the community. Evidently, however, traditional medical-psychiatric services do not adequately fulfill the many needs of these patients. An added complication in managing the middle-aged woman with schizophrenia is that she may have been the primary caregiver for her children and elderly relatives such as her parents. As the primary caregiver for many others, the woman with schizophrenia may herself lack a partner or prime caregiver, so her illness may have severe adverse consequences not only for her but also for her dependents. The advent of community-based treatment may in fact have created more hindrances than assistance for the middle-aged woman with schizophrenia. The fundamental principles for assertive community treatment, as detailed by Stein et al. (1990), have been reproduced by many community intervention workers and consist of the following, modified to emphasize the issues for middle-aged women with psychosis:

1. *An assertive approach.* The lack of motivation for receiving therapy and refusal to accept treatment should not be deterrents in providing care for patients.
2. *Individually tailored programming.* The specific responsibilities and duties of middle-aged women must be fully understood before designing a program—probably one that, to date, has been modeled predominantly on male inpatient populations.
3. *Ongoing monitoring.* This is an important part of assertive treatment, particularly for the middle-aged woman who lacks a designated caregiver, because she may have had the caring role for most of her life.
4. *Tiered support.* Most patients become somewhat dependent on a treatment team, but it is crucial to judge the level of dependency in tandem with the patient's needs, to help her gain maximum independence.
5. *Capitalizing on the patient's strength.* The aim here is to enhance the individual's strengths rather than overemphasize the problems or spend all the time talking about illness.
6. *Crisis resolution availability.* The ability to access crisis teams around the clock is critically important, particularly when there is no clear designated and consistent caregiver. Issues related to domestic violence, homelessness, sexual abuse, comorbid depression, and anxiety may all play a role in managing patients with schizophrenia. However, additional problems may need to be addressed in treating midlife and older women because of the lack of a designated caregiver. Consequently, women may fail to receive prompt attention, or comorbid problems may go unnoticed or relapses be ignored, partly because women tend not to present with violent behavior. Hence, it is vital for clinicians and others to remain alert and identify relapse *signatures* that might otherwise go unnoticed in women patients.

Pharmacological Treatment

Antipsychotic medications are the cornerstone of treatment for schizophrenia and related psychotic disorders. By and large, women with schizophrenia have fewer negative symptoms than men but have more paranoid and delusional symptoms (Goldstein and Tsuang 1990). There are two key features in developing a rational treatment plan for using antipsychotic medication. First, it is essential to recognize the delay between the point at which the patient achieves the desired blood level of an antipsychotic medication and the beginning of clinical improvement. The second point to remember is that once a patient receives an optimal amount of drug, increasing the dose does not lead to a more rapid or greater improvement. Although these principles hold for all patients with schizophrenia, they are often overlooked (Herz and Marder 2002).

In general, antipsychotic drug pharmacodynamics and pharmacokinetics differ by sex and are influenced by body build, diet, smoking, exercise, current medications, substance abuse, and hormones. Women may require lower doses to stay well and may have higher serum levels than men after receiving the same dose. Weight gain, passivity, hypotension, and hyperprolactinemia may be especially problematic in women patients (Seeman 2004).

In deciding what antipsychotic medications to give a woman with a history of schizophrenia as she approaches menopause, the following factors are salient:

- *Subjective response.* The woman's past response to a medication should be assessed.
- *Family history of antipsychotic response.* Because the information from pharmacogenomics shows that treatment responses seem to run in families, in women with a family history of schizophrenia it is vital to find out which medications were successful in treating relatives.
- *Extrapyramidal side effect sensitivity.* Second-generation antipsychotics characteristically produce fewer extrapyramidal side effects, and because extrapyramidal symptoms are serious and disabling drug side effects, the second-generation antipsychotics represent a major advance in antipsychotic drug treatments. If the patient suffers from extrapyramidal side effects, one of the second-generation antipsychotics—especially olanzapine, quetiapine, risperidone, or clozapine—may be the most useful.
- *Tardive dyskinesia.* A review of the literature on gender and tardive dyskinesia shows that some but not all studies identify female sex as a risk factor for developing tardive dyskinesia. A review of cohort studies reveals that tardive dyskinesia is more of a risk factor for older men but that its severity may be greater in older women (Seeman 2004). Studies on the effect of estrogen on tardive dyskinesia are inadequate and have had inconsistent results. Some case reports and small studies have shown an improvement of symptoms in women given estrogen treatment (Bedard et al. 1977; Villeneuve et al. 1978). Glazer et al. (1984) administered 1.25 mg of conjugated estrogens to postmenopausal women with tardive dyskinesia, most of whom had been diagnosed with schizophrenia or schizoaffective disorder, and the movement disorders declined with the addition of estrogen. Given the serious nature of this tardive dyskinesia,

it is important to choose an antipsychotic medication that will not worsen the side effect of tardive dyskinesia and other movement disorders in older women. Drugs such as clozapine, olanzapine, quetiapine, and risperidone appear relatively safer with respect to tardive dyskinesia symptoms. Fewer data are available for ziprasidone and aripiprazole, but early evidence suggests a lower risk of tardive dyskinesia with these drugs as well (Marder et al. 2004).

- *Weight gain.* Around the menopause, many women gain weight; the fat distribution is a particular truncal adipose type. This weight gain is generally attributed to changes in estrogen levels, which affect fat hormone (leptin) metabolism. This weight gain is greatly increased by both typical and atypical antipsychotic drugs. Abnormal weight gain increases the risks of developing type II diabetes, cardiovascular disease, hypertension, stroke, and osteoarthritis (Marder et al. 2004; Nasrallah 2000). In addition, excessive weight and obesity may have deleterious effects on self-image, adjustment in the community, adherence to prescribed medication, and the ability to participate in rehabilitation. If weight gain is a problem in treating schizophrenia, then ziprasidone, risperidone, or quetiapine—medications less associated with weight gain—should be considered (Marder et al. 2004).

- *Impaired glucose metabolism.* Schizophrenia itself may be associated with a higher risk of diabetes mellitus. However, epidemiologic studies show an increased risk of treatment-emergent hyperglycemia-related adverse events in patients treated with several atypical antipsychotics, particularly clozapine and olanzapine. Serious events include ketoacidosis, hyperosmolar coma, and death. Regular glucose control monitoring to identify diabetes mellitus as soon as possible is recommended. U.S. Food and Drug Administration (FDA) warnings for hyperglycemia and diabetes mellitus are now required for clozapine, olanzapine, quetiapine, aripiprazole, risperidone, and ziprasidone.

- *Sedation.* If the woman experiences drug-related lethargy and sedation, then risperidone or aripiprazole may be the medication to use. Of interest is a report that in the elderly, atypical antipsychotics such as quetiapine are metabolized by the enzyme CYP3A4 and that this enzyme may decline with age, resulting in a lower dose requirement for such drugs (Tariot 1999).

- *Cardiovascular disease.* Risks of heart disease are greatly increased by obesity, smoking, diabetes, and a sedentary lifestyle, all of which are fairly common in middle-aged women with schizophrenia. Less common, but nevertheless serious, are the increased risk of pulmonary embolism and cardiac arrhythmias (torsades de pointes because of prolonged QT intervals), both of which are more common in women taking antipsychotic drugs than in men taking these drugs. A number of antipsychotics, including thioridazine, ziprasidone, risperidone, olanzapine, haloperidol, and sertindole, have been found to increase the QT interval (Marder et al. 2004). Emergency use of high-dose intravenous drugs such as haloperidol that prolong the QT interval may be especially dangerous in women (Seeman 2004). In patients with preexisting ischemic heart disease, the use of antipsychotic drugs that induce hypotension should be avoided. Certain antipsychotics can be associated with hyperlipidemias, which may also increase the risk of coronary heart disease. Several reports have found lipid elevation in patients taking atypical antipsychotics, particularly clozapine and olanzapine.

- *Stroke.* FDA warnings have been issued for cerebrovascular adverse events, including strokes and transient ischemic attacks, in older patients taking olanzapine. Consequently, this drug is not approved for patients with dementia-related psychosis.
- *Prolactin elevation.* Women are more prone to drug-induced hyperprolactinemia from atypical antipsychotics than men. Common symptoms related to prolactin elevation in women are decreased libido, infertility, galactorrhea, menstrual irregularities, and poor vaginal lubrication. High prolactin levels decrease bone mineral density and increase the risk of osteoporosis. Women with schizophrenia are already at higher risk for osteoporosis because of low estrogen, poor diet, smoking, lack of exercise, and polydipsia (Seeman 2004). Falls, which may result from drug-induced hypotension, are particularly dangerous in older women with osteoporosis, who are at higher risk for fractures. To avoid hyperprolactinemia, the medications of choice would include olanzapine, quetiapine, ziprasidone, and aripiprazole. Risperidone results in high prolactin levels similar to those of first-generation antipsychotics (Marder et al. 2004).
- *Sexual function.* All antipsychotics may interfere with sexual function. (This may be unrelated to hyperprolactinemia.) Inquiry about the potential side effects will enable tailoring of treatment to increase drug adherence.
- *Cognitive deficit.* For women who have this problem, most of the second-generation antipsychotic drugs may provide moderate benefit.
- *Treatment-resistant positive symptoms.* Clozapine is still regarded as the treatment of choice for treatment-refractory positive symptoms. Patients taking clozapine should be monitored for blood dyscrasias and cardiomyopathy, which are possible side effects.

The second-generation antipsychotics are associated with a range of dose-related side effects, which are different for different medications, and they can also produce idiosyncratic effects such as neuroleptic malignant syndrome. Some of these side effects include hypotension, seizures (with clozapine), extrapyramidal symptoms and prolactin elevation (with risperidone), weight gain and potential increased risk of developing diabetes (with most atypical antipsychotics), and sedation (with quetiapine). For a complete discussion of physical health monitoring of patients with schizophrenia, please see the report of the consensus of psychiatric and other medical experts who evaluated the existing literature and developed recommendations (Marder et al. 2004). It is imperative to understand the individual needs of middle-aged women and to tailor medication to those needs.

Case Example

Sally, a 54-year-old woman, presented with a relapse of psychotic symptoms. She had a 17-year history of auditory hallucinations in which she heard the voices of her family telling her that she was useless. Sally's first episode of illness began after the birth of her third child when she was 37 years old. Since then, she had been treated with 15 mg trifluoperazine per day and her illness had been managed predominantly out of hospital, except for three admissions between the ages of 37 and 50. At age 50, despite no change in antipsychotic medication and no noted psychosocial precipitating factors, Sally described an increase in the frequency and intensity of the auditory hallucinations. She also experienced sleep disturbances and agitation accompanying the psychotic symptomatology. Her treating psychiatrist changed her medication to 15 mg of olanzapine per day, and Sally gained 20 kg during a 6-month period. She was then treated with 6 mg of oral risperidone per day. Two months after this treatment, she developed galactorrhea and described sexual difficulties. At the same time, Sally noted the onset of lip smacking and tardive dyskinesia movements. She was then treated with 300 mg of quetiapine per day and noted great lethargy—which interfered with her ability to parent her teenage children because she was unable to get out of bed until 11:00 A.M. At the same time, Sally described having severe hot flashes (which also interfered with her sleep pattern), increasing facial hirsutism, and irregular periods. Full investigation revealed that Sally had diminished estrogen and progesterone levels and raised FSH levels consistent with menopause. She was successfully treated with 2 mg estradiol plus 10 mg dehydroprogesterone as a continuous preparation and by decreasing the quetiapine to 100 mg twice daily, plus ongoing supportive psychotherapy with her case manager. Today Sally is well and has a good quality of life.

Bipolar Affective Disorder in Women at Perimenopause and Menopause

Unlike unipolar depression, bipolar affective disorder shows no overall difference in prevalence rates between men and women (Kessler et al. 1994). Nevertheless, there are several clinically significant gender-specific differences with respect to this disorder. Women with bipolar disorder are more likely than men to experience depression (Angst 1978) and are at increased risk for rapid cycling (Leibenluft 1996). Women with a history of bipolar disorder appear to experience relapses at low-estrogen phases or exacerbation of the depressive phase in perimenopause (Hendrick et al. 1996).

Of particular interest is the manic phase with psychotic symptoms in women at perimenopause and menopause. Work by Manji and Lenox (1999) suggests that the action of lithium, a potent mood stabilizer, is via protein kinase C inhibition. Manji and Lenox put forward the hypothesis that tamoxifen—which is also a potent protein kinase C inhibitor—may also produce mood stabilization or antimania effects. Being a potent antiestrogenic agent, tamoxifen is believed to have further effects in women via its mood-stabilizing action, particularly for the manic phase of bipolar disorder. In a pilot study (Kulkarni et al. 2003), we found that 40 mg/day of adjunctive tamoxifen relieved manic symptoms in women of childbearing age compared with women receiving only standard lithium treatment. These results seem to support the clinical picture of women with bipolar affective disorder as having more frequent episodes of depression than mania, when they reach menopause and beyond. This concept appears to have some validity, suggesting that lowered estrogen levels may aid in the management of manic symptoms but, as is recognized for depression, may worsen the depressive phase and its associated symptoms. Burt et al. (1998) and Soares and Almeida (2001) described the increased incidence of depression in women during perimenopause, and they advocated a comprehensive assessment of somatic complaints such as vasomotor symptoms (hot flashes and cold sweats) plus careful monitoring of sleep patterns in this age group. In perimenopausal women presenting with depressive symptoms, those given estrogen as therapy found their depressive symptomatology was relieved (Schmidt et al. 2000; Soares et al. 2001). (The management of unipolar depression in perimenopausal and postmenopausal women is discussed in Chapter 4, Mood Disorders, Midlife, and Reproductive Aging.) To date, information about the lifetime prevalence and the clinical picture for midlife and older women suffering from bipolar disorder—in particular the manic phase—is somewhat limited.

Conclusion

The advent of menopause can exert a powerful influence on the lives of women. Whether it is viewed as a stage of liberation or as a loss of childbearing potential, it is undoubtedly a time of extra vulnerability for women predisposed to psychosis. Observations from many different cultures have led to the hypothesis that estrogens are psychoprotective agents (Di Paolo 1994; Fink et al. 1999; Hafner 1991; Seeman 1995). As women approach and reach menopause, there is an increased risk of relapse for those who have schizophrenia and also a risk of new-onset schizophrenia for otherwise healthy women. Therapy for women in perimenopause and thereafter should be holistic, taking into account the psychosocial, biological, and hormonal changes that may well be key driving forces in the emergence of psychotic symptoms or in the exacerbation of existing psychosis. The use of HT is not currently a familiar practice for most mental health clinicians, who may need to remind themselves about all aspects of the whole woman they are managing. Furthermore, the use of antipsychotic and mood-stabilizing medications must be geared to the biological and hormonal changes that play a vital role in drug metabolism. General health issues related to perimenopause and menopause must also be considered in making treatment decisions. As with psychotic disorders in all women, the etiology has biological, psychological, and social components, all of which must be addressed. A woman with schizophrenia may well have experienced cognitive deficits, poor self-esteem, social disabilities, and physical ill health because of her serious mental condition, which can all be exacerbated by menopause. It is imperative that mental health clinicians be aware of and be able to recognize the special problems of women with psychosis as they go through menopause and try to help them attain a good quality of life during this transition period.

References

American Psychiatric Association: Diagnostic and Statistical Manual of Mental Disorders, 4th Edition. Washington, DC, American Psychiatric Association, 1994

Angermeyer MC, Kuhn L, Goldstein JM: Gender and the course of schizophrenia: differences in treated outcomes. Schizophr Bull 116:293–307, 1990

Angst J: The course of affective disorders, II: typology of bipolar manic-depressive illness. Arch Psychiatr Nervenkr 226:65–73, 1978

Baddeley A, Warrington E: Amnesia and the distinction between long and short term memory. Journal of Verbal Learning and Verbal Behavior 9:176–189, 1970

Baddeley A, Logie R, Bressi S, et al: Dementia and working memory. Q J Exp Psychol A 38:603–618, 1986

Baruk H, Melzer R, Vezous A, et al: L'effondremont oestrogenique dans la démence precoce. Étude par la méthode des frottis vaginaux de Papanicolaou. Ann Med Psychol (Paris) 108:181–187, 1950

Bedard P, Langelier P, Villeneuve A: Oestrogens and the extrapyramidal system. Lancet 12:1367–1368, 1977

Bleuler M: Die spätschizophrenen Krankheitsbilder. Fortschr Neurol Psychiatr 15:259–290, 1943

Braendle W, Breckwoldt M, Kuhl H, et al: Sexualhormone und Psyche. Ergebnisse des 2. Interdisziplinären Frankfurter Gesprächs zur Kontrazeption. Frauenarzt 42:154–160, 2001

Burt VK, Altshuler LL, Rasgon N: Depressive symptoms in the perimenopause: prevalence, assessment and guidelines for treatment. Harv Rev Psychiatry 6:121–132, 1998

Ciompi L: The influence of aging on schizophrenia. Triangle 32:25–31, 1993

Clopton J, Gordon JH: In vivo effects of estrogen and 2-hydroxy estradiol on D-2 dopamine receptor agonist affinity states in rat striatum. J Neural Transm 66:13–20, 1986

Davidson L, McGlashan TH: The varied outcomes of schizophrenia. Can J Psychiatry 42:34–43, 1997

Diczfalusy E, Lauritzen C: Oestrogene beim Menschen. Berlin, Springer, 1961

Di Paolo T: Modulation of brain dopamine transmission by sex steroids. Rev Neurosci 5:27–42, 1994

Faraone SV, Chen WJ, Goldstein JM, et al: Gender differences in age at onset of schizophrenia. Br J Psychiatry 164:625–629, 1994

Ferretti C, Blengio M, Vigna I, et al: Effects of estradiol on the ontogenesis of striatal dopamine D_1 and D_2 receptor sites in male and female rats. Brain Res 571:212–217, 1992

Fields JZ, Gordon JH: Estrogen inhibits the dopaminergic supersensitivity induced by neuroleptics. Life Sci 30:229–234, 1982

Fink G, Sumner B, Rosie R, et al: Androgen actions on central serotonin neurotransmission: relevance for mood, mental state and memory. Behav Brain Res 105:53–68, 1999

Glazer WM, Naftolin F, Morgenstern H, et al: Estrogen placement and tardive dyskinesia. Psychoneuroendocrinology 10:345–350, 1984

Goldstein JM, Tsuang MT: Gender and schizophrenia: an introduction and synthesis of findings. Schizophr Bull 16:179–183, 1990

Hafner H: Epidemiology of schizophrenia, in Search for the Causes of Schizophrenia. Edited by Hafner H, Gattaz WF, Janzarik W. Berlin, Springer, 1987, pp 47–74

Hafner H: The epidemiology of beginning schizophrenia. Paper presented at the WPA Section of Epidemiology and Community Psychiatry Symposium, Oslo, June 14–16, 1991

Hafner H, an der Heiden W: Epidemiology of schizophrenia. Can J Psychiatry 42:139–151, 1997

Hendrick V, Altshuler LL, Burt VK: Course of psychiatric disorders across the menstrual cycle. Harv Rev Psychiatry 4:200–207, 1996

Herz M, Marder S: Pharmacologic treatment, in Schizophrenia: Comprehensive Treatment and Management. Edited by Herz M, Marder S. Philadelphia, PA, Lippincott Williams & Wilkins, 2002, pp 73–116

Howard R, Almeida D, Levy R: Phenomenology, demography and diagnosis in late paraphrenia. Psychol Med 24:397–410, 1994

Jeste DV, Harris M, Krull A: Clinical and neuropsychological characteristics of patients with late onset schizophrenia. Am J Psychiatry 152:722–730, 1995

Kessler RC, McGonagle KA, Zhao S, et al: Lifetime and 12-month prevalence of DSM-III-R psychiatric disorders in the United States: results from the National Comorbidity Survey. Arch Gen Psychiatry 51:8–19, 1994

Kraepelin E: Psychiatrie. Bd 1–4. Leipzig, Barth, 1909–1915

Krafft-Ebbing G von: Untersuchungen über Irresein zur Zeit der Menstruation: ein klinischer Beitrag zur Lehre vom periodischen Irresein. Arch Psychiatry 8:65–107, 1896

Kretschmer E: Körperbau und Charakter. Untersuchungen zum Konstitutionsproblem und zur Lehre von den Temperamenten, 25. Berlin, Springer, 1921

Kulkarni J, de Castella A, Smith D, et al: A clinical trial of the effects of estrogen in acutely psychotic women. Schizophr Res 20:247–252, 1996

Kulkarni J, Riedel A, de Castella A, et al: Estrogen: a potential treatment for schizophrenia. Schizophr Res 48:137–144, 2001

Kulkarni J, de Castella A, Downey M, et al: Results of two controlled studies on estrogen: avenue to neuroprotection in schizophrenia, in Risk and Protective Factors in Schizophrenia. Edited by Hafner H. Darmstadt, Germany, Steinkopff Verlag, 2002, pp 271–282

Kulkarni J, Scaffidi A, de Castella A, et al: Antiestrogens: a potential treatment in bipolar affective disorder? Paper presented at the International Congress on Schizophrenia Research, Colorado Springs, CO, May 2003

Leibenluft E: Women with bipolar illness: clinical and research issues. Am J Psychiatry 153:163–173, 1996

Mall G: Diagnostik und Therapie ovarieller Psychosen. Zentralblatt für die gesamte Neurologie und Psychiatrie 155:250, 1960

Manji HK, Lenox RH: Protein kinase C signaling in the brain: molecular transduction of mood stabilization in the treatment of manic-depressive illness. Biol Psychiatry 46:1328–1351, 1999

Marder SR, Essock SM, Miller AL, et al: Physical health monitoring of patients with schizophrenia. Am J Psychiatry 161:1334–1349, 2004

Mason P, Harrison G, Glazebrook G, et al: The characteristics of outcome in schizophrenia at 13 years. Br J Psychiatry 167:596–603, 1995

Milner B: Disorders of learning and memory after temporal lobe lesions in man. Clin Neurosurg 19:421–446, 1972

Nasrallah H: High prevalence of diabetes mellitus in schizophrenia, schizoaffective disorder, and bipolar disorder (abstract P.01.096). Int J Neuropsychopharmacol 3 (suppl 1):S116, 2000

Opjordsmoen S: Long-term clinical outcome of schizophrenia with special reference to gender differences. Acta Psychiatr Scand 83:307–313, 1991

Pearlson G, Rabins P: Late-onset psychoses: the possible risk factors. Psychiatr Clin North Am 11:15–32, 1988

Riecher-Rossler A, Loffler W, Munk-Jorgensen P: What do we really know about late-onset schizophrenia? Eur Arch Psychiatry Clin Neurosci 247:195–208, 1997

Schmidt PJ, Nieman L, Danaceau MA, et al: Estrogen replacement in perimenopause-related depression: a preliminary report. Am J Obstet Gynecol 183:414–420, 2000

Seeman MV: Gender differences in schizophrenia. Can J Psychiatry 27:107–112, 1982

Seeman MV: Sex differences in predicting neuroleptic response, in The Prediction of Neuroleptic Response. Edited by Gaebel W, Awad AG. Vienna, Springer-Verlag 1995, pp 51–64

Seeman MV: Does menopause intensify symptoms in schizophrenia? in Psychiatric Illness in Women. Edited by Lewis Hall F, Williams T, Panetta J, et al. Washington, DC, American Psychiatric Publishing, 2002, pp 239–248

Seeman MV: Gender differences in the prescribing of antipsychotic drugs. Am J Psychiatry 161:1324–1333, 2004

Sherwin B: Estrogen and cognitive functioning in women. Endocr Rev 24:133–151, 2003

Soares CN, Almeida OP: Depression during the perimenopause (letter). Arch Gen Psychiatry 58:306, 2001

Soares CN, Almeida OP, Joffe H, et al: Efficacy of estradiol for the treatment of depressive disorders in perimenopausal women: a double-blind, randomized, placebo-controlled trial. Arch Gen Psychiatry 58:529–534, 2001

Stein LI, Diamond RJ, Factor RM: A system approach to the care of persons with schizophrenia, in Handbook of Schizophrenia, Vol IV. Edited by Herz MI, Keith SJ, Docherty JP, et al. New York, Elsevier, 1990, pp 213–246

Steinmeyer EM, Marneros A, Deister A, et al: Long-term outcome of schizoaffective and schizophrenic disorders: a comparative study, II: causal-analytical investigations. Eur Arch Psychiatry Clin Neurosci 238:126–134, 1989

Tariot PN: The older patient: the ongoing challenge of efficacy and tolerability. J Clin Psychol 60 (suppl 23):29–33, 1999

Tulving E: Episodic and semantic memory, in Organization of Memory. Edited by Tulving E, Donaldson W. New York, Academic Press, 1972, pp 381–403

Villeneuve A, Langelier P, Bedard P: Estrogens, dopamine and dyskinesias. Can Psychiatr Assoc J 23:68–70, 1978

Wong DF, Wagner HN Jr, Dannals RF, et al: Effects of age on dopamine and serotonin receptors measured by positron emission tomography in the living human brain. Science 226:1393–1396, 1984

Wykes T, Parr AM, Landau S: Group treatment of auditory hallucinations. Exploratory study of effectiveness. Br J Psychiatry 175:180–185, 1999

Chapter 6

Medical Aspects of Perimenopause and Menopause

Angela M. Cheung, M.D., Ph.D., F.R.C.P.C.

*M*enopause has traditionally been considered a transition in life. From a medical perspective, women often move into a period of increased risk for various medical conditions. Among postmenopausal women, the most frequent causes of mortality in North America are cardiovascular diseases (American Heart Association 2003; Mosca et al. 1997) and cancer (American Cancer Society 2004). Breast cancer, lung cancer, and colorectal cancer account for the greatest proportion of cancer deaths in this group (American Cancer Society 2004). The major causes of morbidity and disability are osteoporotic fractures, arthritis, and dementia (Chaudhry and Cheung 2002; Cheung et al. 2003). Thyroid diseases are also common but have less associated morbidity or mortality (Schindler 2003). These conditions can be detected as early as in the perimenopausal period, but they are more commonly observed in the postmenopausal period, often 10–20 years after menopause. Although the onset and progression of these conditions are associated with aging, decreased levels of female hormones with menopause and the use of hormone therapy (HT) also have an impact on them. This chapter focuses on how menopause and HT can affect these conditions and highlights important recent findings in these areas.

Hormone Therapy

Hormone therapy (unopposed estrogen or combined estrogen plus progestin therapy) is effective in relieving perimenopausal symptoms such as hot flashes, urogenital disorders, and sleep disturbance, and estrogen may be beneficial for mood changes in some women (Cardozo et al. 1998; Ginsburg 1994; Zweifel and O'Brien 1997). See Chapter 4, Mood Disorders, Midlife, and Reproductive Aging. In recent decades, interest and controversy have arisen regarding the use of HT for the prevention of chronic diseases. Currently, both estrogen and progestin are available in a variety of types (estrogen: estradiol, conjugated equine estrogen [CEE], estrone, and estropipate; progestin: medroxyprogesterone acetate [MPA], norethindrone acetate, and micronized progestin) and formulations (oral pills, topical creams, and patches). With the emergence of data showing an increased risk of endometrial cancer, the use of unopposed estrogen alone in women with natural menopause has declined in recent years. For women in whom HT is indicated, current recommendations for a woman with an intact uterus are to use both estrogen and progestin to decrease the risk of endometrial cancer, and to use progestin for a period of at least 10–14 days every 1–3 months (North American Menopause Society 2003). For a woman without a uterus, estrogen alone can be used. The U.S. Food and Drug Administration (FDA) advises that estrogen and progestin therapy be used at the lowest dose possible for the shortest duration possible.

Women's Health Initiative

The Women's Health Initiative (WHI) is a large multicenter observational and interventional primary prevention study that recruited 161,809 postmenopausal women between 1993 and 1998 (Women's Health Initiative Study Group 1998). Various arms of the study are examining the effects of low dietary fat, calcium and vitamin D supplementation, and hormone use. The two arms of the study involving hormone use, one with combined estrogen plus progestin therapy involving 16,608 women with an intact uterus (Writing Group for the Women's Health Initiative Investigators 2002), and the other with estrogen-only therapy involving 10,739 women with hysterectomy (Women's Health Initiative Steering Committee 2004), were both terminated prematurely in May 2003 and February 2004, respectively. They were double-blind, placebo-controlled, randomized trials. The primary end points were coronary artery disease, stroke, and invasive breast cancer. Other end points included venous thromboembolic events, hip fractures, colon cancer, endometrial cancer, and cognition and quality of life. The combined estrogen plus progestin therapy trial had an average follow-up of 5.2 years and involved postmenopausal women with a mean age of 63.3 years at entry to the study: 5,522 were ages 50–59 years, 7,510 were 60–69 years, and 3,576 were 70–79 years. Most (*n*=12,304) had never been exposed to HT prior to study entry; a small proportion of women were past users (*n*=3,262) and current users (*n*=1,035). The estrogen-only therapy trial had an average follow-up of 6.8 years and involved women with a mean age of 63.6 years at entry. The demographic characteristics of the population are similar to those in the other arm.

Results from these two arms of the study have generated significant interest, concern, and controversy and will be discussed in the disease-specific sections in this chapter. These trials are not perfect, and there is ongoing debate about the ramifications of their methodologic limitations. The majority of women in these trials started HT many years after menopause, and some critics have questioned whether the effect will be similar for those who have been on HT since menopause. These trials addressed two types of HT (one dosing regimen for each), and some have wondered if other types or doses would have similar effects. There were also compliance and follow-up issues in the trials. Also, some have questioned whether the observed increased risk of cardiovascular disease with hormone use could be a result of detection bias, because two or more letters went out to participants warning them of a slightly increased risk of cardiovascular events occurring in the first year or so after starting therapy. Despite all these methodologic limitations, the WHI trials are the largest to date examining prevention of chronic diseases with HT in the postmenopausal population, and we do need to consider their findings and those of other recent studies when giving advice to patients with regard to HT (Table 6–1).

Cardiovascular Disease

Cardiovascular disease is the leading cause of death among postmenopausal women in North America (American Heart Association 2003; Mosca et al. 1997). The term is a broad one that encompasses coronary artery disease, peripheral vascular disease, valvular heart disease, congestive heart failure, hypertension, and arrhythmia. Coronary artery disease is by far the largest component of cardiovascular disease, and the impact of menopause on cor-

TABLE 6–1. Annual rates of events prevented or caused per 10,000 women taking combined estrogen-progestin or estrogen-only hormone therapy (HT) versus placebo

Outcome	Combined estrogen-progestin HT		Estrogen-only HT	
	Prevented	Caused	Prevented	Caused
Cardiovascular disease events				
Coronary artery disease events	—	7[a]	—	—
Stroke	—	8[a]	—	12[b]
Thromboembolism	—	18[a]	—	7[b]
Total	—	25[a]	—	24[b]
Cancer				
Breast (invasive)	—	8[a]	—	—
Ovarian	—	—	—	2[c]
Colorectal	6[a]	—	—	—
Cholecystitis				
<5 yr therapy or placebo use	—	25[d]	—	—
≥5 yr therapy or placebo use	—	53.5[d]	—	—
Fracture				
Hip	5[a]	—	6[b]	—
Vertebra	6[a]	—	6[b]	—
Other (including wrist)	39[a]	—	—	—
Total	44[a]	—	56[b]	—

Note. This table is meant as a guide for discussion with patients; an individual's risk profile may alter the balance of harms and benefits.

[a]These data are from the Women's Health Initiative (WHI) estrogen-plus-progestin trial (Manson 2003; Writing Group for the Women's Health Initiative Investigators 2002), in which the HT regimen was the daily combination of oral conjugated equine estrogen (0.625 mg) and medroxyprogesterone acetate (2.5 mg).

[b]These data are from the WHI estrogen-only trial, in which the daily estrogen-only HT regimen was oral conjugated equine estrogen (0.625 mg).

[c]These data are from Lacey et al. 2002.

[d]These data are from the systematic review and meta-analysis by Nelson et al. (2002).

Source. Adapted from Wathen et al. 2004.

onary artery disease is one of the most studied areas. The Framingham Heart Study, a prospective cohort study that started in the 1960s, showed that post-menopausal women are at significantly increased risk of cardiovascular events as compared with premenopausal women at the same age (Gordon et al. 1978; Kannel et al. 1976). The Nurses' Health Study, another large-scale prospective cohort study in the United States, showed that current estrogen users were less likely than past users, who in turn were less likely than never users, to have cardiovascular disease (Stampfer et al. 1991; Wilson et al. 1985). Research has also shown that the risk of developing heart disease is greater after surgical menopause than with natural menopause, especially when the surgery is done before the age of natural menopause (Eaker et al. 1993).

There have been many hypotheses regarding the role of estrogen in the pathogenesis of atherosclerosis (Mendelsohn et al. 2000, 2002; Samaan and Crawford 1995). Estrogen has been postulated to affect the development or progression of factors that increase the risk of atherosclerosis, such as hyper-cholesterolemia, diabetes, and hypertension. The Postmenopausal Estrogen/Progestin Interventions (PEPI) Trial, a double-blind, placebo-controlled, randomized trial, involved 875 postmenopausal women and examined the effects of four different oral hormone regimens on lipid profiles: unopposed CEE, combined CEE and cyclical MPA, daily combined CEE and MPA, and daily combined CEE and micronized progestin (Writing Group for the PEPI Trial 1995). At the end of 3 years, they found that all hormonal regimens had beneficial effects on lipid profile when compared with placebo. Among the hormone groups, the unopposed-CEE group had the best profile (increasing the high-density lipoprotein [HDL] cholesterol the most), and the daily combined CEE+MPA group had the worst profile. Using the same population, researchers were able to show that HT moderately decreased fasting levels of insulin and glucose (Espeland et al. 1998; Fineberg 2000). Similarly, Kanaya and colleagues (2003) were also able to demonstrate that HT reduced the incidence of diabetes by 35% in women with coronary disease. Previous studies have observed increases in blood pressure with menopause and a beneficial reduction of blood pressure with estrogen therapy (Wyss and Carlson 2003). One suggested means by which estrogen affects blood pressure is by decreasing sympathetic nervous system activity (Meyer et al. 2001; Vongpatanasin et al. 2001). Most physiologic studies in postmenopausal women have shown beneficial effects of estrogen therapy on blood pressure, although randomized controlled trials have shown conflicting results (Affinito et al. 2001; Cacciatore et al. 2001; De Meersman et al. 1998; Harvey et al. 1999, 2000; Hayward et al. 2001; Manwaring et al. 2000; Scuteri et al. 2001a).

Estrogen has also been postulated to have effects on other cardiovascular risk factors, such as homocysteine (Barnabei et al. 1999) and C-reactive protein (Cushman et al. 1999), and to have direct vessel effects (Gorodeski et al. 1998; Kawecka-Jaszcz et al. 2002; Scuteri et al. 2001b; Sung et al. 1999). Research from the PEPI Trial showed that estrogen decreased homocysteine levels and increased levels of C-reactive protein (an inflammation-sensitive protein that has recently been found to be a marker of cardiovascular disease). Estrogen was also found to decrease levels of E-selectin (another inflammation-sensitive protein), which are modulated by polymorphism of the estrogen receptor α (Cushman et al. 1999; Herrington et al. 2002). Although animal studies have shown that estrogen decreases plaque formation, increases vasodilation, and has antiproliferation and antioxidant effects, clinical trials in postmenopausal women have been less promising. Herrington et al. (2000) examined the effects of estrogen therapy on the progression of coronary artery atherosclerosis in 309 postmenopausal women in the Estrogen Replacement and Atherosclerosis trial. After an average of 3.2 years' follow-up, they found that neither CEE alone nor CEE+MPA affected the progression of coronary atherosclerosis in women with established disease as determined by quantitative coronary angiography. Herrington and colleagues (2001) also analyzed brachial artery flow-mediated vasodilation in 1,662 postmenopausal women in the Cardiovascular Health Study, a longitudinal study of cardiovascular risk factors in subjects over 65 years of age. They did not find overall differences in brachial flow-mediated vasodilator responses between hormone users and nonusers, even after adjusting for potential confounds. This lack of effect was most noted in women over age 80 and in those with established cardiovascular disease. However, among women without clinical or subclinical cardiovascular disease or its risk factors, there was a significant association between use of HT and flow-mediated vasodilator responses.

Despite promising effects of HT on cholesterol, glycemic control, and blood pressure, large studies of HT in recent years have shown disappointing results in "hard" outcomes such as myocardial infarction, revascularization, and hospitalization for acute coronary syndrome. The WHI combined CEE+MPA arm showed a 29% increase in coronary heart disease in the hormone group compared with placebo after an average of 5.2 years of follow-up (Writing Group for the Women's Health Initiative Investigators 2002). This increase in cardiovascular events began in the first year of use and continued throughout the study. Although the WHI recruited postmenopausal women in the general population, the Heart and Estrogen/progestin Replacement Study (HERS) specifically recruited postmenopausal women with cardiovascular disease (Hulley et al. 1998). This randomized, double-blind, placebo-controlled trial involved 2,763 postmenopausal women and examined the effects of combined CEE+MPA on cardiovascular outcomes. At the end of 4.1 years of average follow-up, HT did not decrease the risk of cardiovascular events. In fact, there was a trend toward more cardiovascular events in the hormone group in the first 2 years. An open-label extension to this study (HERS II) involving 2,321 postmenopausal women for an average of 2.7 years also did not show a decrease in cardiovascular events with HT (Grady et al. 2002). Because of results of these studies, the American Heart Association (Mosca et al. 2001) and the North American Menopause Society (2003) are currently recommending against using HT as first-line therapy for the primary or secondary prevention of cardiovascular disease in postmenopausal women. These recommendations have stayed in place even after the discontinuation of the WHI estrogen-only arm, which showed no increased cardiovascular risks with estrogen only in postmenopausal women with hysterectomy (Women's Health Initiative Steering Committee 2004). This is because the estrogen-only arm failed to demonstrate a beneficial effect on cardiovascular outcomes after an average of 6.8 years of follow-up.

Stroke

Stroke is the third leading cause of death and a leading cause of disability in North American women (American Heart Association 2003). Major risk factors for stroke include atrial fibrillation, hypertension, diabetes mellitus, smoking, and hyperlipidemia. The prevalence of risk factors for stroke is similar among women and men, although postmenopausal women are more likely to have a diagnosis of hypertension and less likely to be smoking. The incidence of stroke increases with age, and the loss of estrogen around menopause may increase that risk by increasing the prevalence of hypertension and diabetes.

Current randomized controlled trials have not shown a protective effect of HT on the risk of stroke. The HERS did not show a difference between the hormone and placebo groups in terms of progression of carotid atherosclerosis as measured by the temporal change in intimal medial thickness (Byington et al. 2002). The Women's Estrogen for Stroke Trial (WEST), a prospective, double-blind, placebo-controlled, randomized trial of estradiol 1 mg/day versus placebo in 664 postmenopausal women with recent stroke or transient ischemic attacks, found no overall decrease in the risk of stroke or stroke death in an average of 2.8 years of follow-up (Viscoli et al. 2001). In fact, the investigators found a two- to threefold increase in the risk of stroke in the first 6 months. More recently, the combined CEE+MPA arm of the WHI Study showed a 41% increase in strokes in the hormone group compared with the placebo group (Writing Group for the Women's Health Initiative Investigators 2002). This increased risk appeared to be present in all subgroups of women, not just those at high risk for strokes (Wassertheil-Smoller et al. 2003). The estrogen-only arm of the WHI Study also showed a 39% increase in strokes in the hormone group (Women's Health Initiative Steering Committee 2004). Thus, HT is currently not recommended for the primary or secondary prevention of stroke.

Cancer

Breast Cancer

Breast cancer accounts for approximately one-third of all new cancers diagnosed in women in North America (American Cancer Society 2004). Over the past decade, the incidence of breast cancer has increased steadily, although the mortality rates for breast cancer have declined. The risk of developing breast cancer increases with age, positive family history of breast cancer (especially in a first-degree relative who developed it at a young age), early menarche, late menopause, low parity, older age at first pregnancy, higher weight, previous radiation exposure, previous benign breast disease, use of HT, and a high-fat diet. Some of these risk factors, such as early menarche, late menopause, higher weight, and use of HT, relate to total lifetime estrogen exposure.

The use of HT has been shown to increase the risk of developing breast cancer in postmenopausal women in both observational cohort studies (Colditz et al. 1993; Dupont and Page 1991; Grady et al. 1992; Sillero-Arenas et al. 1992; Steinberg et al. 1991) and randomized controlled trials (Writing Group for the Women's Health Initiative Investigators 2002). The meta-analysis performed by the Collaborative Group on Hormonal Factors in Breast Cancer (1997) reanalyzed the primary data from 47 studies (32 case-control, 15 prospective cohort) and included 17,949 women with breast cancer and 35,916 women without breast cancer in their analyses. They showed a 14% increase in breast cancer risk in women who were ever users compared with those who were never users. More recently, the Million Women Study, a population-based cohort study of 800,000 women ages 50–64 years in the United Kingdom, also showed that women who were using HT were 1.66 times more likely than women who never used HT to develop breast cancer and 1.22 times more likely to die from it (Million Women Study Collaborators 2003).

In fact, researchers have consistently observed an increase in risk with duration of use (Colditz et al. 1993; Collaborative Group on Hormonal Factors in Breast Cancer 1997; Grady et al. 1992; Sillero-Arenas et al. 1992; Steinberg et al. 1991). This increased risk was often not observed until after 5 or more years of use. In the Collaborative Group study, current users and those who had used HT within the past 4 years experienced a 2.3% increase in risk for each additional year of use (Collaborative Group on Hormonal Factors in Breast Cancer 1997). The WHI combined CEE+MPA arm exhibited a 26% increase in the risk of invasive breast cancer in the hormone group, especially after 4 years of use (Writing Group for the Women's Health Initiative Investigators 2002), whereas the estrogen-only arm did not show an increased risk after an average follow-up of 6.8 years (Women's Health Initiative Steering Committee 2004). Many researchers have postulated that the formulation of the HT, in terms of the type and dose of estrogen and progestin used, may modulate this risk increase. Whether the type of estrogen used affects the risk of breast cancer is controversial (Bergkvist et al. 1989; Collaborative Group on Hormonal Factors in Breast Cancer 1997; Hulka et al. 1982). However, over the past few years there has been increasing evidence from the Swedish cohort in Uppsala Province, the U.S. Breast Cancer Detection Demonstration Project, and the Million Women Study to suggest that combination therapy with progestin increases breast cancer risk beyond that of estrogen alone (Million Women Study Collaborators 2003; Persson et al. 1999; Schairer et al. 2000; Women's Health Initiative Steering Committee 2004).

Lung Cancer

Lung cancer is the leading cause of cancer death among women in North America (American Cancer Society 2004). In general, it is divided into two histologic subtypes: small cell lung cancer and non–small cell lung cancer. Small cell lung cancer is a rapidly progressing form with a poor prognosis and is seen in approximately 25% of lung cancer patients. The non–small cell group is further divided into squamous cell carcinoma and adenocarcinoma (Simmonds 1999). Women who smoke are at higher risk of developing small cell lung cancer than non–small cell lung cancer (Baldini et al. 1997). Women smokers who develop non–small cell lung cancer are more likely to have adenocarcinoma than squamous cell carcinoma (Ferguson et al. 1990).

Approximately 90% of lung cancer deaths in men and women are associated with cigarette smoking and are therefore considered preventable. The remaining 10% of lung cancer deaths occur in nonsmokers who are mainly women (Stabile and Siegfried 2003). For over a decade, mortality rates have increased at a rate of approximately 2.5% per year in women, a direct correlate of increased smoking and increased exposure to secondhand smoke among women (American Cancer Society 2004). Among women, approximately 90% of all lung cancer cases are diagnosed in those 50 years or older, and close to half are diagnosed in those 70 years or older.

It is only recently that researchers and clinicians have paid attention to the effect of estrogen on lung cancer in women (Siegfried 2001). In animal models, estrogen played a role in lung carcinogenesis (Jiang et al. 2000). Recently, researchers discovered that human non–small cell lung cancer cells and cells derived from normal lung expressed estrogen receptors (both the α and β types) and responded to estrogen stimulation (Stabile et al. 2002). Evidence from a number of epidemiologic studies suggests that women are more sensitive than men to the effects of tobacco smoke (Harris et al. 1993; Risch et al. 1993; Zang and Wynder 1996). Two Chinese studies and one Swedish study have shown that lung cancer risk is related to hormonal status in women (Adami et al. 1989; Gao et al. 1987; Liao et al. 1996). Early age at menopause has been shown to decrease the risk of adenocarcinoma of the lung, whereas the use of HT is associated with a higher risk of adenocarcinoma of the lung (Stabile and Siegfried 2003). There is also a positive relationship among HT, smoking, and the development of adenocarcinoma of the lung (Taioli and Wynder 1994). Women who smoked cigarettes and received estrogen therapy were at 32.4 times the risk of developing adenocarcinoma of the lung as women who never smoked who were taking estrogens. These results suggest that estrogen may promote lung cancer and that blocking the effects of estrogen could potentially stop disease progression or prevent its recurrence.

Colorectal Cancer

Colorectal cancer is the third leading cause of cancer among women in North America (American Cancer Society 2004). Rates for colorectal cancer have declined significantly in the past decade. However, the number of new cases continues to rise because the population is aging, and the incidence of colorectal cancer increases with age. Two meta-analyses have shown that estrogen modulates the occurrence of colorectal cancer (Grodstein et al. 1999; Nanda et al. 1999). The first one, by Grodstein and colleagues (1999), found a 20% decrease in colon cancer risk and a 19% decrease in rectal cancer risk among ever users of HT when compared with never users. Current users appeared to have a greater risk reduction (34% relative risk reduction). There were no significant effects observed for the duration, type, and dosage of estrogen use or the addition of progestin. The second meta-analysis showed that it was the recency of hormone use, and not merely past use, that conferred the decreased risk of developing colon cancer (Nanda et al. 1999). Moreover, researchers have observed that longer duration of hormone use was associated with decreased risk of colon cancer. The WHI combined CEE+MPA trial is the first randomized controlled trial to demonstrate a significantly decreased risk of colorectal cancer (37% relative risk reduction) with combination HT, even though this was not one of their primary end points (Writing Group for the Women's Health Initiative Investigators 2002).

Osteoporosis

Osteoporosis affects one in five postmenopausal women in North America (National Osteoporosis Foundation 2004). A group of experts convened by the World Health Organization (WHO) in 1993 defined *osteoporosis* as a disease characterized by low bone mass and microarchitectural deterioration of bone tissue, resulting in bone fragility and an increased risk of fractures ("Consensus Development Conference" 1993). In 2001, an expert panel convened by the National Institutes of Health amended the definition of *bone strength* to include both bone density and bone quality ("Osteoporosis Prevention, Diagnosis, and Therapy" 2000). Osteoporosis is asymptomatic until a fracture occurs. The most significant impact of osteoporosis is osteoporotic fractures. These fractures, particularly of the hip and spine, cause considerable morbidity and mortality. On average, a 50-year-old woman's lifetime risk of a forearm fracture is 16%; spine fracture, 15.6%; hip fracture, 17.5%; and any osteoporotic fracture, greater than 40% (Melton et al. 1992). Postmenopausal women who have sustained multiple vertebral fractures can develop spine deformity, which can lead to restrictive lung disease (Leech et al. 1990), early satiety, chronic pain, and low self-esteem (Nevitt et al. 2000). Even radiographic vertebral fractures (asymptomatic vertebral deformities that are diagnosed only on X rays) are associated with decreased quality of life (Adachi et al. 2001), increased hospitalization, and increased mortality (Ensrud et al. 2000). Those with hip fractures have pain, decreased mobility, fear of falling, and loss of independence (Cauley et al. 2000; Greendale et al. 1995; Wiktorowicz et al. 2001). As many as 20% of hip fracture patients will die in their first year postfracture, often because of complications arising from hospitalization (Cooper et al. 1993). Both hip and vertebral fractures are associated with similarly decreased 5-year survival (Cauley et al. 2000). Whether the decrease in survival can be attributed to fractures or to comorbid illnesses is controversial (Kado et al. 1999).

The key risk factors for osteoporotic fractures are increasing age, low body mass index, a history of previous fracture, and low bone mineral density (BMD) (Cheung et al. 2004). A relationship between BMD and fracture risk has been observed in a number of studies, and BMD remains the best quantifiable predictor of osteoporotic fracture for those who have not had a fragility fracture. The standard classification for osteoporosis and osteopenia is based on the 1993 WHO criteria, which compare BMD to that of a reference population of postmenopausal Caucasian women (Kanis and WHO Study Group 1994). Using the WHO criteria, a BMD value greater than or equal to 2.5 standard deviations below the young adult mean is defined as osteoporosis, and a BMD value between 1 and 2.5 standard deviations below the young adult mean is defined as osteopenia. Women with osteopenia have a lower risk of fracture than women with osteoporosis, but they may be at greater risk than women with normal BMD. The prevalence of osteopenia among women age 50 or over in North America is approximately 50% (Looker et al. 1997).

Postmenopausal women are at increased risk for this disease because the loss of estrogen causes more resorption than formation in the bone remodeling cycle. In the first 5 years immediately after menopause, women can experience bone loss at a rate of 2%–5% per year. This rate of bone loss usually diminishes after about 10 years, to 1%–2% per year. Previous studies have shown that HT increases bone density and reduces fractures (Grady et al. 1992; Torgerson and Bell-Syer 2001). The WHI Study has shown that combined CEE+MPA reduces hip fractures by 34% and total fractures by 24%, but the number of women who would have to be treated to prevent one event is huge (Writing Group for the Women's Health Initiative Investigators 2002). Even when we examine all the pros and cons of using HT in postmenopausal osteoporotic women, the risks outweigh the benefits (Cauley et al. 2003). Thus, multiple scientific and medical bodies, such as the U.S. Preventive Services Task Force (2002), the North American Menopause Society (2003), and the American College of Obstetricians and Gynecologists (2002), have recommended against the use of HT as first-line therapy for the treatment and prevention of osteoporosis since the release of the WHI results. It has also been shown that HT does not have a sustained effect on BMD. Once HT is discontinued, the rate of bone loss can return to perimenopausal or early menopausal levels, especially in the first 2 years (Bone et al. 2000; Greendale et al. 2002; Greenspan et al. 2002; Neele et al. 2002; Tremollieres et al. 2001). For a woman with osteoporosis, switching to another osteoporosis therapy when coming off hormones is recommended (see later for details; Cheung et al. 2004). For those without osteoporosis (those with normal BMD or with osteopenia) who are at low risk for fractures, regular monitoring of BMD is recommended.

Osteoporotic fractures place a substantial burden on postmenopausal women, their social supports, and the health care system because these fractures often result in loss of independence and decreased quality of life. An understanding of factors that contribute to fractures, and of strategies to prevent falls, is important, especially in decreasing hip fractures among elderly persons. Prevention and treatment can be started early in women at high risk for fracture. Preventive strategies currently include lifestyle modifications, such as ensuring adequate dietary calcium and vitamin D intake, increasing physical activity or exercise, smoking cessation, and reducing caffeine intake and alcohol intake. Pharmacological treatment options include bisphosphonates and selective estrogen receptor modulators (SERMs). Parathyroid hormone, calcitonin, and HT may be used in selected cases, although the risks may outweigh the benefits in the case of HT. Dietary supplements should be used in women who cannot obtain adequate dietary calcium and vitamin D (current recommendations for postmenopausal women are 1,500 mg of calcium and 800 IU of vitamin D per day). Weight-bearing exercise can increase peak bone mass in teenagers and help maintain bone mass in postmenopausal women. Non-weight-bearing exercises, such as yoga, tai chi, and Pilates, can improve balance and reduce falls. For women who are prone to falls, wearing hip protectors can reduce the risk of hip fractures (Lauritzen et al. 1993). Environmental adaptations such as having handrails in bathrooms and bathtubs, having night-lights to improve night vision, and eliminating loose rugs and slippery surfaces in and around the home are important as well in fall prevention.

Arthritis

Arthritis is a general term that encompasses a wide range of joint disorders, including those resulting from degenerative disease, inflammatory disease, and posttraumatic damage. The most common form is osteoarthritis, a degenerative disorder characterized by destruction and loss of cartilage and damage to underlying bone. Rheumatoid arthritis, a systemic autoimmune disease, is less common than osteoarthritis. There are no known cures for any form of arthritis, and for the most part the underlying causes are not well understood. As a result, arthritis tends to be chronic and progressive and is the leading cause of long-term disability and health care utilization (Badley et al. 1995; Guccione et al. 1994; Reynolds et al. 1992; Williams et al. 1998). In North America, it is also the second leading cause for taking prescription and over-the-counter medications and the third leading cause for consulting a health professional (Williams et al. 1998). Arthritis affects more women than men, and prevalence increases with age. The prevalence ranges from 22% (for women ages 45–54) to 56% (for women age 75 or older) (Badley and Wang 1998; Dunlop et al. 2001). In the Women's Health and Aging Study, a survey of disabled, community-dwelling women, the investigators found arthritis to be the most commonly reported chronic condition among disabled, community-dwelling women age 65 or older (Hochberg et al. 1995).

The impact of loss of estrogen associated with menopause and the impact of use of HT has been studied in arthritis patients (Wluka et al. 2000). A number of studies have shown that pregnancy exacerbates disease activity in systemic lupus erythematosus and ameliorates disease activity in rheumatoid arthritis (Cutolo et al. 2002a, 2002b; Doria et al. 2002; Kanik and Wilder 2000; Khamashta et al. 1997; Kiss et al. 2002; Ostensen 1999). The role of female hormones in rheumatoid arthritis is one of the most studied areas of immunomodulation by estrogen (Bijlsma 1999; Druckmann 2001). Whether HT decreases disease activity and the risk of developing rheumatoid arthritis in postmenopausal women is controversial (Barrett-Connor

1999; Cutolo 2002; Cutolo et al. 2002a, 2002b; Hall et al. 1994; Koepsell et al. 1994; MacDonald et al. 1994; van den Brink et al. 1993). Randomized controlled trials have failed to demonstrate a beneficial effect of HT on disease activity in postmenopausal women with rheumatoid arthritis. Bone loss and osteoporosis are hallmarks of rheumatoid arthritis (Bijlsma and Jacobs 2000; Gough et al. 1994; Iwamoto et al. 2002; Kroger et al. 1994; Shenstone et al. 1994; Shibuya et al. 2002). The Oslo-Truro-Amsterdam Collaborative Study showed that women with rheumatoid arthritis often have low BMD and vertebral deformities and that radiographically documented damage secondary to rheumatoid arthritis is correlated with the degree of low BMD and the number of vertebral deformities (Lodder et al. 2003). The use of hormone therapy in these women may decrease bone loss and prevent osteoporosis, especially in those using corticosteroid therapy (Hall et al. 1993)—although the risks associated with HT may outweigh its benefits even in this population.

It is only in recent years that researchers have paid more attention to the role of estrogen in osteoarthritis (Cooley et al. 2003; Felson and Nevitt 1998; Richette et al. 2003; Tsai and Liu 1992). Estrogen receptors can be found in human cartilage, and a variant of the estrogen receptor gene is a genetic marker for generalized osteoarthritis (Ushiyama et al. 1998). Although HT has been demonstrated to reduce the severity of osteoarthritis in animal models (Ham et al. 2002), studies in humans have yielded conflicting results (Dennison et al. 1998; Nevitt and Felson 1996; Reginster et al. 2003). There are no randomized controlled trials designed to specifically assess the effect of HT on symptomatic or structural progression of osteoarthritis. Large-scale observational studies and trials designed to assess other potential benefits of estrogens suggest that HT does not provide symptomatic relief in osteoarthritis, but it may decrease long-term structural progression, particularly in the lower limbs (Barrett-Connor 1999; Erb et al. 2000; Felson 1990; Nevitt et al. 2001; Spector et al. 1997; Wluka et al. 2001).

Dementia

Alzheimer's disease, the most common cause of dementia, is a progressive neurodegenerative condition characterized by cognitive impairment and overall functional decline. Alzheimer's disease is responsible for approximately two-thirds of dementia cases and is more common in women than in men (Goa et al. 1998; Jorm and Jolley 1998). Vascular dementia, a condition caused by systemic vascular disease such as atherosclerosis and hypertension, is the second most common form of dementia. It is responsible for approximately 20% of dementia cases and is more common in men. Incidence increases with age, especially after age 85 (Canadian Study of Health and Aging Working Group 2000; Goa et al. 1998; Rockwood and Stadnyk 1994). A number of studies have shown that the survival of women with dementia is much poorer than that of women without cognitive impairment (Koutsavlis and Wolfson 2000). Women diagnosed with Alzheimer's disease or vascular dementia have a 5-year mortality rate of close to 60% in the 65–74 age group, and greater than 80% in the 85 and older age group. Women ages 65–74 years with dementia have 10 times the risk of death at 5 years compared with women of the same age in the general population, and women age 85 or older with dementia have twice the risk of death compared with same-age women in the general population (Ostbye et al. 1999).

Mild cognitive impairment is a recently described syndrome that is thought of as a transition phase between healthy cognitive aging and dementia. The definition of *mild cognitive impairment* varies (Fisk et al. 2003), but it usually implies subjective complaint of memory impairment, and objective memory impairment when adjusted for age and education, in the absence of dementia (Petersen et al. 1999). It is thought to affect 3%–4% of nondemented persons age 65 or over in the general population (Ganguli et al. 2004). Although 7%–20% of women with mild cognitive impairment converted to Alzheimer's disease per year (Johnson et al. 1998; Petersen et al. 1999; Wolf et al. 1998), a substantial proportion also remained stable or reverted to normal over a 10-year follow-up period (Ganguli et al. 2004). In general, women diagnosed with cognitive impairment other than vascular dementia or Alzheimer's disease have a better prognosis but still fare worse than the general population. Most dementias are progressive and irreversible. The social and financial impact on families and society is very large (Hux et al. 1998).

Increasing age, a positive family history, and a low level of education are known to be significant risk factors for Alzheimer's disease. There are data to suggest that the loss of estrogen has a negative impact on cognitive impairment around menopause (for details, see Chapter 3, Effects of Reproductive Hormones and Selective Estrogen Receptor Modulators on the Central Nervous System During Menopause), but there is still controversy about whether the use of estrogen therapy is protective against dementia, especially Alzheimer's disease. Although a number of observational studies suggest that women who take estrogen preserve or even improve their cognitive function more than women who do not, there are also a number of studies that do not support this hypothesis (Benson 1999; Birge 1996; McBee et al. 1997; Yaffe et al. 1998). In a meta-analysis, LeBlanc and colleagues (2001) found a 34% relative risk reduction in hormone users, but they indicated that the variability in interventions, measures, and design and quality of the individual studies makes it difficult to draw strong conclusions. Also, the results need to be interpreted with caution because of the lack of random assignment and a possible "healthy user bias" in the observational studies. The best evidence to date in this area is the Women's Health Initiative Memory Study, which is part of the two hormone arms of the WHI Study (Rapp et al. 2003; Shumaker et al. 2003, 2004). This substudy included 4,532 postmenopausal women in the combined CEE+MPA arm and 2,947 women in the CEE-only arm. It showed that HT (either combined CEE+MPA or CEE only) increased the risk of dementia and mild cognitive impairment by about 40% in postmenopausal women age 65 years or older, after an average of 4.5 years of follow-up (Shumaker et al. 2004).

Thyroid Disease

Hypothyroidism is common in postmenopausal women. In a population of postmenopausal women, 2.4% were found to have overt thyroid disease, and 23% had subclinical thyroid disease (Schindler 2003). In the latter group, 74% were hypothyroid, and 26% were hyperthyroid. The vast majority of cases of hypothyroidism are the result of a primary thyroid disorder such as primary idiopathic hypothyroidism, ablation of the thyroid by radioactive iodine treatment, thyroidectomy, or Hashimoto's thyroiditis.

The symptoms of hypothyroidism may be mistakenly ascribed to menopause or depression. Clinicians should be alert to the possibility of thyroid disease in women presenting with complaints such as fatigue, apathy, weight gain, mood change, memory loss, or cognitive impairment. In extreme cases, severe untreated hypothyroidism can result in confusion, coma, or even death. Hypothyroidism is also associated with an increased risk of cardiovascular events because of increased total cholesterol, increased low-density lipoprotein (LDL) cholesterol, and decreased levels of HDL cholesterol.

Hypothyroidism can be easily treated with daily oral levothyroxine. The goal of therapy is to achieve a euthyroid state, as demonstrated by thyroid-stimulating hormone (TSH) levels in the normal range. Hypothyroidism should usually be corrected gradually, especially in patients who are elderly or are known to have coronary artery disease. In these individuals, a sudden increase in metabolic rate may precipitate cardiac ischemia, even at a dose of thyroid hormone that would normally maintain a euthyroid state. In patients with impaired cognitive function or mood changes, improvement may not be seen until weeks to months after levothyroxine therapy has been instituted.

There is significant controversy as to whether thyroid replacement therapy causes decreased bone density. If untreated for prolonged periods, hyperthyroidism can certainly increase bone turnover and decrease bone density, especially in postmenopausal women. However, levothyroxine therapy for hypothyroidism does not increase the risk of osteoporosis if TSH levels are properly maintained in the normal range.

Recent data suggest that estrogen plays a role in regulating thyroid hormone requirements. In women with hypothyroidism who are started on estrogen therapy, thyroxine requirements may increase (Arafah 2001). In a group of 25 postmenopausal women with hypothyroidism treated with thyroxine, the institution of estrogen therapy resulted in decreased serum free thyroxine and increased serum TSH. These alterations were likely a result of estrogen-induced increases in serum thyroxine-binding globulin concentration. The results from this study also suggest that women with hypothyroidism may require less thyroxine supplementation when they go through menopause. In addition, thyroxine requirements typically decrease with aging. Therefore, routine screening of thyroid function with TSH to detect subclinical thyroid disease around the time of menopause is recommended.

Other Effects of Menopause or Hormone Use

Hormone therapy increases the risk of thromboembolic diseases, such as deep vein thrombosis and pulmonary embolism, in postmenopausal women (Grady et al. 2000; Miller et al. 2002; Writing Group for the Women's Health Initiative Investigators 2002). The mechanism for this is unclear, although many have postulated this is a result of estrogen modulation of the coagulation system. In both the HERS and the WHI Study, postmenopausal women on combined CEE+MPA therapy were found to be at twice to three times the risk for thromboembolic events (Grady et al. 2000; Writing Group for the Women's Health Initiative Investigators 2002). Hormone therapy also increased the risk of cholecystitis in the first 5 years of use by 80% and by two- to threefold with sustained use (Grodstein et al. 1994). Although previous observational studies have shown an association of less urinary incontinence with hormone use, more recent data from the HERS have disputed this claim (Grady et al. 2001). Grady and colleagues found that daily combined oral estrogen plus progestin therapy was associated with worsening urinary incontinence in older postmenopausal women with weekly incontinence. See also Chapter 7 in this volume, Gynecologic Aspects of Perimenopause and Menopause.

Many perimenopausal and postmenopausal women are treated with HT by their health care providers to improve quality of life. However, data from the combined HT arm of the WHI Study showed that HT did not improve health-related quality of life in the overall study population (Hays et al. 2003). In the subgroup of women with perimenopausal or postmenopausal symptoms, a larger proportion of women on HT had improvement in the severity of hot flashes and the severity of night sweats compared with women on placebo at 1 year; however, other than a small improvement in sleep disturbance, there was no difference in health-related quality of life. This surprising finding is one more reason for us to reevaluate our rationale for prescribing HT to postmenopausal women who are asymptomatic.

Current Guidelines for Hormone Therapy

Our current knowledge has several limitations that must be considered when counseling patients. The evidence presented within this chapter applies to the prevention of chronic diseases, not menopausal symptoms (which are addressed in Chapter 7, Gynecologic Aspects of Perimenopause and Menopause). The results of the combined estrogen and progestin trial and the estrogen-only trial in the WHI and many of the observational studies apply to a specific drug regimen (CEE 0.625 mg/day plus MPA 2.5 mg) and may not necessarily apply to other formulations of oral estrogens and progestins. However, there are no data to suggest that other combinations are different. Alternative preparations of HT will need to undergo rigorous testing before their long-term safety can be determined. With the discontinuation of the combined estrogen plus progestin arm of the WHI Study, a large primary prevention trial in the United Kingdom, the Women's International Study of Long Duration Oestrogen After Menopause was also stopped (Medical Research Council 2002). More recently, the estrogen-only arm of the WHI Study was also stopped prematurely.

On the basis of current evidence, the U.S. Preventive Services Task Force (2002), North American Menopause Society (2003), American College of Obstetricians and Gynecologists (2002), and the FDA (U.S. Food and Drug Administration 2003) have all recommended against using the daily combined estrogen and progestin therapy for the prevention of chronic diseases. The FDA has extended the warning that HT causes more harm than benefit to all estrogen preparations, including oral and transdermal forms, and to both estrogen-only and combined estrogen plus progestin. Most other scientific bodies either have suggested not using unopposed estrogen for the prevention of chronic diseases until further evidence to support its use is available or have refrained from issuing a recommendation for or against its use. For the treatment of menopausal symptoms such as vasomotor symptoms and atrophic vaginitis, all have suggested using as low a dose as possible for as short a duration as possible. The use of HT should be reviewed periodically to assess whether it is still required. See also Chapter 7, Gynecologic Aspects of Perimenopause and Menopause.

New Therapies

The many new therapies that are specific to the various disease areas are beyond the scope of this chapter. Of note, there is a new class of compounds called selective estrogen receptor modulators (SERMs). See also Chapter 3, Effects of Reproductive Hormones and Selective Estrogen Receptor Modulators on the Central Nervous System During Menopause, and Chapter 7, Gynecologic Aspects of Perimenopause and Menopause. These compounds are very different from estrogens in structure and function, and they can be broadly grouped in two classes, triphenylethylenes and benzothiophenes. The oldest marketed agent is tamoxifen, which belongs to the triphenylethylene class. Tamoxifen has been used as adjuvant therapy for breast cancer and, more recently, for the prevention of breast cancer in high-risk women. Because it increases the risk of endometrial cancer and endometrial hyperplasia, it is not a feasible option as preventive therapy for chronic diseases.

A newer compound belonging to the benzothiophene class, called raloxifene, is marketed for the prevention and treatment of osteoporosis. It is often considered a second-generation SERM, with tamoxifen belonging to the first generation. In primary prevention trials, raloxifene has been shown to result in modest increases in BMD. The Multiple Outcomes of Raloxifene Evaluation (MORE) is a multicenter, double-blind, placebo-controlled, randomized trial involving 7,705 postmenopausal women with osteoporosis and an average age of 65 years (Ettinger et al. 1999). After 3 years of follow-up, postmenopausal osteoporotic women without previous vertebral fractures had a 55% relative risk reduction on raloxifene, whereas those with previous vertebral fractures had a 30% relative risk reduction. These magnitudes of risk reduction are comparable to those for bisphosphonates (Black et al. 1996; Cummings et al. 1998; Harris et al. 1999; Reginster et al. 2000). Among postmenopausal women with osteoporosis, the risk of invasive breast cancer was decreased by 76% during 3 years of treatment with raloxifene (Cummings et al. 1999).

In terms of cardiovascular risk factors, raloxifene has been shown to be similar to estrogen with respect to improving lipid profiles (except that it does not increase HDL cholesterol or triglycerides) and endothelial function and decreasing fibrinogen, Lp(a) lipoprotein, and homocysteine levels (Anderson et al. 2001; Saitta et al. 2001; Walsh et al. 1998, 2000). It has been shown to decrease C-reactive protein, whereas estrogen has been shown to increase it (Walsh et al. 2001). Because of the concern about HT's increasing the risk of cardiovascular diseases, researchers from the MORE trial also did post hoc analyses to determine the effect of raloxifene on cardiovascular outcomes. Overall, in this osteoporotic group, there was no difference between raloxifene and placebo in terms of cardiovascular outcomes, and no observed increased risk in the first 1 or 2 years (Barrett-Connor et al. 2002). In a high-risk subgroup, as defined by a history of coronary disease or having risk factors for coronary disease, researchers were able to demonstrate a protective effect of raloxifene on overall cardiovascular outcomes (40% relative risk reduction) and stroke (72% relative risk reduction).

There are several large-scale ongoing studies examining cardiovascular and breast outcomes with raloxifene. The Raloxifene Use for the Heart trial involving 10,101 postmenopausal women is expected to have results in another 3–5 years. The Continuous Outcomes of Raloxifene Evaluation trial, a continuation of the MORE trial, examining breast cancer as the primary outcome, has been completed, and results are expected to be released soon. Recruitment has been completed for the Study of Tamoxifen and Raloxifene for the prevention of breast cancer, which involves approximately 19,000 women. Other than raloxifene, there are several other SERMs in development, and some are in the planning phases for Phase III clinical trials.

Relevance to Mental Health

Postmenopausal women are at increased risk for developing various medical conditions, some of which have been highlighted in this chapter. The link between mental health and some of these conditions is complex. On one hand, women with depression are at increased risk for some of these conditions. Recent data suggest that depression increases the risks of first myocardial infarction and cardiovascular mortality by a factor of 1.5–2 (Todaro et al. 2003; Wulsin and Singal 2003) and stroke by a factor of 1.3–2.6 (Jonas and Mussolino 2000; Ohira et al. 2001; Ostir et al. 2001; Robinson 2003). On the other hand, these medical conditions can increase a woman's risk of developing psychological and psychiatric problems, the most common of which is depression. The prevalence of major depression has been estimated to range from 15% to 23% among those with coronary disease (Burg and Abrams 2001) and from 13% to 26% among those with cancer (Chochinov 2001; Chochinov et al. 1994; Derogatis et al. 1983; Hjerl et al. 2002; Massie and Popkin 1998). Among individuals with strokes, major depression is common, especially in women (Berg et al. 2001, 2003; Burvill et al. 1995; Kotila et al. 1998), and the increase in incidence persists many years after the initial insult (Astrom et al. 1993; Dam 2001; Sharpe et al. 1990; Wilkinson et al. 1997). Moreover, those with medical conditions and comorbid depression tend to do worse, have lower rehabilitation potential, and have higher associated morbidity and mortality (Barefoot et al. 1996; Carney and Freedland 2002; Hjerl et al. 2003; Horsten et al. 2000; House et al. 2001;

Popovich et al. 2002; Ramasubbu and Patten 2003; Rigler 1999).

The diagnosis and treatment phases of an acute medical illness are often stressful. Besides depression, they can induce posttraumatic stress disorder in some (Green et al. 1998; Smith et al. 1999) and panic disorder in others (Fleet et al. 1998). These illnesses often come at a time when there is little or no social or financial support. Women may be widowed and may have an attrition of friends because of death. These factors can compound the situation and increase the risk of depression for those who are predisposed. Although feeling sad is a normal reaction to the many fears, anxieties, and uncertainties associated with the diagnosis of medical conditions in the postmenopausal period, major depression is a serious psychiatric disorder that can affect many of these women, causing additional suffering. Depression is often underrecognized and undertreated in women with medical conditions, especially those with recent myocardial infarctions or acute stroke. On depression associated with menopause, see Chapter 3, Effects of Reproductive Hormones and Selective Estrogen Receptor Modulators on the Central Nervous System During Menopause, and Chapter 4, Mood Disorders, Midlife, and Reproductive Aging.

In the past, there have been concerns about certain antidepressants causing adverse outcomes in patients with medical conditions—for example, tricyclic antidepressants in coronary patients. Over the past decade, there have been a number of double-blind, placebo-controlled, randomized trials on the use of selective serotonin reuptake inhibitors in patients with acute myocardial infarctions, stroke, and cancer. The Sertraline AntiDepressant Heart Attack Randomized Trial found that 6-month treatment with sertraline was both safe and effective for treating major depression in the immediate period after hospitalization for acute coronary syndrome (Glassman et al. 2002; Swenson et al. 2003). Sertraline did not affect left ventricular ejection fraction or QTc interval, and it did not increase ventricular premature complex runs or other cardiovascular adverse events. Several trials have also demonstrated that fluoxetine is effective in treating poststroke depression (Fruehwald et al. 2003; Wiart et al. 2000). Another study showed that treatment with fluoxetine or nortriptyline for 12 weeks during the first 6 months poststroke significantly increased the survival of both depressed and nondepressed patients over a 9-year follow-up period (Jorge et al. 2003). This finding raises more questions about the intricate links between the mind and the body, and suggests that the increased mortality associated with certain medical conditions may be modifiable by antidepressants. Because of their tolerability and effectiveness, selective serotonin reuptake inhibitors have become the preferred class of antidepressants for the treatment of clinically depressed medical patients, although choice of therapy should be individualized.

TABLE 6–2. Preventive procedures recommended for postmenopausal women by the U.S. Preventive Services Task Force

Interventions	Age group	Frequency	Level of recommendation	Date updated
Screening				
Cardiovascular				
Blood pressure	All	Yearly	A	2003
Lipids	Age ≥ 45	Yearly	A	2001
Cancer				
Mammogram with or without clinical breast exam	Age ≥ 40	Every 1–2 years	B	2002
Pap smears	Age ≤ 65	Every ≤ 3 years	A	2003
Fecal occult blood tests	Age ≥ 50	Yearly	A	2002
Osteoporosis and fractures				
BMD test	Age ≥ 65	Every 2 years	B	2002
Others				
BMI	All	Yearly	B	2003
Depression	All	Periodically	B	2002
Alcohol misuse	All	Periodically	B	2004
Vision (Snellen acuity test)	All	Periodically	B	1996
Hearing (question regarding problem)	Older adults	Periodically	B	1996

TABLE 6–2. Preventive procedures recommended for postmenopausal women by the U.S. Preventive Services Task Force *(continued)*

Interventions	Age group	Frequency	Level of recommendation	Date updated
Immunizations				
Pneumococcal vaccine	Age≥65	Every 5–10 years	B	1996
Influenza vaccine	Age≥age 65	Yearly	B	1996
Tetanus-diphtheria boosters	All	Every 10 years	A	1996
Counseling				
Smoking cessation	All	Periodically	A	2003
Fall prevention	Elderly	Periodically	B	1996
Motor vehicle injuries	All	Periodically	B	1996
–Use of seatbelts	All	Periodically	B	1996
–Avoidance of alcohol and drugs	All	Periodically	B	1996

Note. BMD=bone mineral density; BMI=body mass index.

Source. Adapted for postmenopausal women from the U.S. Preventive Services Task Force Recommendations for the General Population (U.S. Preventive Services Task Force 1996, 2000).

The recognition of the relationship between the medical aspects of menopause and mental health is important for mental health practitioners as well as medical specialists. Encouraging preventive health practices in depressed postmenopausal women is important for reducing the risk of acquiring medical conditions (Table 6–2). Early identification of depression among those with medical conditions can lead to effective therapeutic intervention and better outcome. The good news is that the incidence of depression in women is lowest in the postmenopausal period (Kessler et al. 2003). With good prevention, treatment, and coping strategies, postmenopausal women can reduce the risks of increased morbidity and mortality associated with menopause and aging. Life after menopause can be highly productive, functional, and enjoyable. Mental health practitioners have an important role to play in improving quality of life in perimenopausal and postmenopausal women.

References

Adachi JD, Ioannidis G, Berger C, et al: The influence of osteoporotic fractures on health-related quality of life in community-dwelling men and women across Canada. Osteoporos Int 12:903–908, 2001

Adami HO, Persson I, Hoover R, et al: Risk of cancer in women receiving hormone replacement therapy. Int J Cancer 44:833–839, 1989

Affinito P, Palomba S, Bonifacio M, et al: Effects of hormonal replacement therapy in postmenopausal hypertensive patients. Maturitas 40:75–83, 2001

American Cancer Society: Cancer Facts and Figures 2004. Publ No 5008.04. Atlanta, GA, American Cancer Society, 2004

American College of Obstetricians and Gynecologists: Questions and answers on hormone therapy. ACOG News Release August 2002. Available at: http://www.acog.org/from_home/publications/press _release/nr08–30–02.cfm. Accessed December 15, 2003.

American Heart Association: Heart Disease and Stroke Statistics: 2004 Update (Publ No 55–0575). Dallas, TX, American Heart Association, 2003

Anderson PW, Cox DA, Sashegyi A, et al: Effects of raloxifene and hormone replacement therapy on markers of serum atherogenicity in healthy postmenopausal women. Maturitas 39:71–77, 2001

Arafah BM: Increased need for thyroxine in women with hypothyroidism during estrogen therapy. N Engl J Med 344:1743–1749, 2001

Astrom M, Adolfsson R, Asplund K: Major depression in stroke patients: a 3-year longitudinal study. Stroke 24:976–982, 1993

Badley EM, Wang PP: Arthritis and the aging population: projections of arthritis prevalence in Canada 1991–2031. J Rheumatol 25:138–144, 1998

Badley EM, Webster GK, Rasooly I: The impact of musculoskeletal disorders in the population: are they aches and pains? Findings from the 1990 Ontario Health Survey. J Rheumatol 22:733–739, 1995

Baldini EH, Strauss GM: Women and lung cancer: waiting to exhale. Chest 112 (suppl 4):229S–234S, 1997

Barefoot JC, Helms MJ, Mark DB, et al: Depression and long-term mortality risk in patients with coronary artery disease. Am J Cardiol 78:613–617, 1996

Barnabei VM, Phillips TM, Hsia J: Plasma homocysteine in women taking hormone replacement therapy: the Postmenopausal Estrogen/Progestin Interventions (PEPI) Trial. J Womens Health Gend Based Med 8:1167–1172, 1999

Barrett-Connor E: Postmenopausal estrogen therapy and selected (less-often-considered) disease outcomes. Menopause 6:14–20, 1999

Barrett-Connor E, Grady D, Sashegyi A, et al: Raloxifene and cardiovascular events in osteoporotic postmenopausal women: four-year results from the MORE (Multiple Outcomes of Raloxifene Evaluation) randomized trial. MORE investigators. JAMA 287:847–857, 2002

Benson S: Hormone replacement therapy and Alzheimer's disease: an update on the issues. Health Care Women Int 20:619–638, 1999

Berg A, Palomaki H, Lehtihalmes M, et al: Poststroke depression in acute phase after stroke. Cerebrovasc Dis 12:14–20, 2001

Berg A, Palomaki H, Lehtihalmes M, et al: Poststroke depression: an 18-month follow-up. Stroke 34:138–143, 2003

Bergkvist L, Adami HO, Persson I, et al: The risk of breast cancer after estrogen and estrogen-progestin replacement. N Engl J Med 321:293–297, 1989

Bijlsma JW: Can we use steroid hormones to immunomodulate rheumatic diseases? Rheumatoid arthritis as an example. Ann N Y Acad Sci 876:366–377, 1999

Bijlsma JW, Jacobs JW: Hormonal preservation of bone in rheumatoid arthritis. Rheum Dis Clin North Am 26:897–910, 2000

Birge SJ: Is there a role for estrogen replacement therapy in the prevention and treatment of dementia? J Am Geriatr Soc 44:865–870, 1996

Black DM, Cummings SR, Karpf DB, et al: Randomised trial of effect of alendronate on risk of fracture in women with existing vertebral fractures. Fracture Intervention Trial Research Group. Lancet 348:1535–1541, 1996

Bone HG, Greenspan SL, McKeever C, et al: Alendronate and estrogen effects in postmenopausal women with low bone mineral density. Alendronate/Estrogen Study Group. J Clin Endocrinol Metab 85:720–726, 2000

Burg MM, Abrams D: Depression in chronic medical illness: the case of coronary heart disease. J Clin Psychol 57:1323–1337, 2001

Burvill PW, Johnson GA, Jamrozik KD, et al: Prevalence of depression after stroke: the Perth Community Stroke Study. Br J Psychiatry 166:320–327, 1995

Byington RP, Furberg CD, Herrington DM, et al: Effect of estrogen plus progestin on progression of carotid atherosclerosis in postmenopausal women with heart disease: HERS B-mode substudy. Heart and Estrogen/progestin Replacement Study Research Group. Arterioscler Thromb Vasc Biol 22:1692–1697, 2002

Cacciatore B, Paakkari I, Hasselblatt R, et al: Randomized comparison between orally and transdermally administered hormone replacement therapy regimens of long-term effects on 24-hour ambulatory blood pressure in postmenopausal women. Am J Obstet Gynecol 184:904–909, 2001

Canadian Study of Health and Aging Working Group: The incidence of dementia in Canada. Neurology 55:66–73, 2000

Cardozo L, Bachmann G, McClish D, et al: Meta-analysis of estrogen therapy in the management of urogenital atrophy in postmenopausal women: second report of the Hormones and Urogenital Therapy Committee. Obstet Gynecol 92:722–727, 1998

Carney RM, Freedland KE: Psychological distress as a risk factor for stroke-related mortality. Stroke 33:5–6, 2002

Cauley JA, Thompson DE, Ensrud KC, et al: Risk of mortality following clinical fractures. Osteoporos Int 11:556–561, 2000

Cauley JA, Robbins J, Chen Z, et al: Effects of estrogen plus progestin on risk of fracture and bone mineral density: the Women's Health Initiative randomized trial. Women's Health Initiative Investigators. JAMA 290:1729–1738, 2003

Chaudhry R, Cheung AM: Postmenopausal/senior women, in Ontario Women's Health Status Report. Edited by Stewart DE, Cheung AM, Ferris LE, et al. Toronto, ON, Women's Health Council, 2002, pp 314–337

Cheung AM, Chaudhry R, Kapral M, et al: Perimenopausal and postmenopausal health, in Women's Health Surveillance Report: A Multidimensional Look at the Health of Canadian Women. Edited by DesMeules M, Stewart DE. Toronto, ON, Canadian Institute for Health Information, 2003, pp 47–48

Cheung AM, Feig D, Kapral M, et al: Prevention of osteoporosis and osteoporotic fractures in postmenopausal women: recommendation statement from the Canadian Task Force on Preventive Health Care. CMAJ 170:1665–1667, 2004

Chochinov HM: Depression in cancer patients. Lancet Oncol 2:499–505, 2001

Chochinov HM, Wilson KG, Enns M, et al: Prevalence of depression in the terminally ill: effects of diagnostic criteria and symptom threshold judgments. Am J Psychiatry 151:537–540, 1994

Colditz GA, Egan KM, Stampfer MJ: Hormone replacement therapy and risk of breast cancer: results from epidemiologic studies. Am J Obstet Gynecol 168:1473–1480, 1993

Collaborative Group on Hormonal Factors in Breast Cancer: Breast cancer and hormone replacement therapy: collaborative reanalysis of data from 51 epidemiological studies of 52,705 women with breast cancer and 108,411 women without breast cancer. Lancet 350:1047–1059, 1997

Consensus Development Conference: diagnosis, prophylaxis, and treatment of osteoporosis. Am J Med 94:646–650, 1993

Cooley HM, Stankovich J, Jones G, et al: The association between hormonal and reproductive factors and hand osteoarthritis. Maturitas 45:257–265, 2003

Cooper C, Atkinson EJ, Jacobsen SJ, et al: Population-based study of survival after osteoporotic fractures. Am J Epidemiol 137:1001–1005, 1993

Cummings SR, Black DM, Thompson DE, et al: Effect of alendronate on risk of fracture in women with low bone density but without vertebral fractures: results from the Fracture Intervention Trial. JAMA 280:2077–2082, 1998

Cummings SR, Eckert S, Krueger KA, et al: The effect of raloxifene on risk of breast cancer in postmenopausal women: results from the MORE (Multiple Outcomes of Raloxifene Evaluation) randomized trial. JAMA 281:2189–2197, 1999

Cushman M, Legault C, Barrett-Connor E, et al: Effect of postmenopausal hormones on inflammation-sensitive proteins: the Postmenopausal Estrogen/Progestin Interventions (PEPI) Study. Circulation 100:717–722, 1999

Cutolo M: Sex hormone adjuvanting therapy in rheumatoid arthritis. Lupus 11:670–674, 2002

Cutolo M, Seriolo B, Villaggio B, et al: Androgens and estrogens modulate the immune and inflammatory responses in rheumatoid arthritis. Ann N Y Acad Sci 966:131–142, 2002a

Cutolo M, Villaggio B, Craviotto C, et al: Sex hormones and rheumatoid arthritis. Autoimmun Rev 1:284–289, 2002b

Dam H: Depression in stroke patients 7 years following stroke. Acta Psychiatr Scand 103:287–293, 2001

De Meersman RE, Zion AS, Giardina EG, et al: Estrogen replacement, vascular distensibility, and blood pressures in postmenopausal women. Am J Physiol 274:H1539–H1544, 1998

Dennison EM, Arden NK, Kellingray S, et al: Hormone replacement therapy, other reproductive variables and symptomatic hip osteoarthritis in elderly white women: a case-control study. Br J Rheumatol 37:1198–1202, 1998

Derogatis LR, Morrow GR, Fetting J, et al: The prevalence of psychiatric disorders among cancer patients. JAMA 249:751–757, 1983

Doria A, Cutolo M, Ghirardello A, et al: Steroid hormones and disease activity during pregnancy in systemic lupus erythematosus. Arthritis Rheum 47:202–209, 2002

Druckmann R: Review: female sex hormones, autoimmune diseases and immune response. Gynecol Endocrinol 15 (suppl 6):69–76, 2001

Dunlop DD, Manheim LM, Song J, et al: Arthritis prevalence and activity limitations in older adults. Arthritis Rheum 44:212–221, 2001

Dupont WD, Page DL: Menopausal estrogen replacement therapy and breast cancer. Arch Intern Med 151:67–72, 1991

Eaker ED, Chesebro JH, Sacks FM, et al: Cardiovascular disease in women. Circulation 88:1999–2009, 1993

Ensrud KE, Thompson DE, Cauley JA, et al: Prevalent vertebral deformities predict mortality and hospitalization in older women with low bone mass. J Am Geriatr Soc 48:241–249, 2000

Erb A, Brenner H, Gunther KP, et al: Hormone replacement therapy and patterns of osteoarthritis: baseline data from the Ulm Osteoarthritis Study. Ann Rheum Dis 59:105–109, 2000

Espeland MA, Hogan PE, Fineberg SE, et al: Effect of postmenopausal hormone therapy on glucose and insulin concentrations. PEPI Investigators. Postmenopausal Estrogen/Progestin Interventions. Diabetes Care 21:1589–1595, 1998

Ettinger B, Black DM, Mitlak BH, et al: Reduction of vertebral fracture risk in postmenopausal women with osteoporosis treated with raloxifene: results from a 3-year randomized clinical trial. Multiple Outcomes of Raloxifene Evaluation (MORE) Investigators. JAMA 282:637–645, 1999

Felson DT: The epidemiology of knee osteoarthritis: results from the Framingham Osteoarthritis Study. Semin Arthritis Rheum 20 (3 suppl 1):42–50, 1990

Felson DT, Nevitt MC: The effects of estrogen on osteoarthritis. Curr Opin Rheumatol 10:269–272, 1998

Ferguson MK, Skosey C, Hoffman PC, et al: Sex-associated differences in presentation and survival in patients with lung cancer. J Clin Oncol 8:1402–1407, 1990

Fineberg SE: Glycaemic control and hormone replacement therapy: implications of the Postmenopausal Estrogen/Progestogen Intervention (PEPI) Study. Drugs Aging 17:453–461, 2000

Fisk JD, Merry HR, Rockwood K: Variations in case definition affect prevalence but not outcomes of mild cognitive impairment. Neurology 61:1179–1184, 2003

Fleet RP, Dupuis G, Marchand A, et al: Panic disorder in coronary artery disease patients with noncardiac chest pain. J Psychosom Res 44:81–90, 1998

Fruehwald S, Gatterbauer E, Rehak P, et al: Early fluoxetine treatment of post-stroke depression: a 3-month double-blind placebo-controlled study with an open-label long-term follow up. J Neurol 250:347–351, 2003

Ganguli M, Dodge HH, Shen C, et al: Mild cognitive impairment, amnestic type: an epidemiologic study. Neurology 63:115–121, 2004

Gao Y, Blot WJ, Zheng W, et al: Lung cancer among Chinese women. Int J Cancer 40:604–609, 1987

Ginsburg ES: Hot flashes: physiology, hormonal therapy, and alternative therapies. Obstet Gynecol Clin North Am 21:381–390, 1994

Glassman AH, O'Connor CM, Califf RM, et al: Sertraline treatment of major depression in patients with acute MI or unstable angina. JAMA 288:701–709, 2002

Goa S, Hendrie HC, Hall KS, et al: The relationships between age, sex, and the incidence of dementia and Alzheimer's disease. Arch Gen Psychiatry 55:809–815, 1998

Gordon T, Kannel WB, Hjortland MC, et al: Menopause and coronary heart disease: the Framingham Study. Ann Intern Med 89:157–161, 1978

Gorodeski GI, Yang T, Levy MN, et al: Modulation of coronary vascular resistance in female rabbits by estrogen and progesterone. J Soc Gynecol Investig 5:197–202, 1998

Gough AK, Lilley J, Eyre S, et al: Generalised bone loss in patients with early rheumatoid arthritis. Lancet 344:23–27, 1994

Grady D, Rubin SM, Petitti DB, et al: Hormone therapy to prevent disease and prolong life in postmenopausal women. Ann Intern Med 117:1016–1037, 1992

Grady D, Wenger NK, Herrington D, et al: Postmenopausal hormone therapy increases risk for venous thromboembolic disease. The Heart and Estrogen/progestin Replacement Study. Ann Intern Med 132:689–696, 2000

Grady D, Brown JS, Vittinghoff E, et al: Postmenopausal hormones and incontinence: the Heart and Estrogen/progestin Replacement Study. HERS Research Group. Obstet Gynecol 97:116–120, 2001

Grady D, Herrington D, Bittner V, et al: Cardiovascular disease outcomes during 6.8 years of hormone therapy: Heart and Estrogen/progestin Replacement Study follow-up (HERS II). HERS Research Group. JAMA 288:49–57, 2002

Green BL, Rowland JH, Krupnick JL, et al: Prevalence of posttraumatic stress disorder in women with breast cancer. Psychosomatics 39:102–111, 1998

Greendale GA, Barrett-Connor E, Ingles S, et al: Late physical activity and functional effects of osteoporotic fracture: the Rancho Bernardo Study. J Am Geriatr Soc 43:955–961, 1995

Greendale GA, Espeland M, Slone S, et al: Bone mass response to discontinuation of long-term hormone replacement therapy: results from the Postmenopausal Estrogen/Progestin Interventions (PEPI) Safety Follow-up Study. PEPI Safety Follow-up Study (PSFS) Investigators. Arch Intern Med 162:665–672, 2002

Greenspan SL, Emkey RD, Bone HG, et al: Significant differential effects of alendronate, estrogen, or combination therapy on the rate of bone loss after discontinuation of treatment of postmenopausal osteoporosis: a randomized, double-blind, placebo-controlled trial. Ann Intern Med 137:875–883, 2002

Grodstein F, Colditz GA, Stampfer MJ: Postmenopausal hormone use and cholecystectomy in a large prospective study. Obstet Gynecol 83:5–11, 1994

Grodstein F, Newcomb PA, Stampfer MJ: Postmenopausal hormone therapy and the risk of colorectal cancer: a review and meta-analysis. Am J Med 106:574–582, 1999

Guccione AA, Felson DT, Anderson JJ, et al: The effects of specific medical conditions on the functional limitations of elders in the Framingham Study. Am J Public Health 84:351–358, 1994

Hall GM, Spector TD, Griffin AJ: The effect of rheumatoid arthritis and steroid therapy on bone density in postmenopausal women. Arthritis Rheum 36:1510–1516, 1993

Hall GM, Daniels M, Huskisson EC, et al: A randomised controlled trial of the effect of hormone replacement therapy on disease activity in postmenopausal rheumatoid arthritis. Ann Rheum Dis 53:112–116, 1994

Ham KD, Loeser RF, Lindgren BR, et al: Effects of long-term estrogen replacement therapy on osteoarthritis severity in cynomolgus monkeys. Arthritis Rheum 46:1956–1964, 2002

Harris RE, Zang EA, Anderson JI, et al: Race and sex differences in lung cancer risk associated with cigarette smoking. Int J Epidemiol 22:592–599, 1993

Harris ST, Watts NB, Genant HK, et al: Effects of risedronate treatment on vertebral and nonvertebral fractures in women with postmenopausal osteoporosis: a randomized controlled trial. Vertebral Efficacy With Risedronate Therapy (VERT) Study Group. JAMA 282:1344–1352, 1999

Harvey PJ, Wing LM, Savage J, et al: The effects of different types and doses of oestrogen replacement therapy on clinic and ambulatory blood pressure and the renin-angiotensin system in normotensive postmenopausal women. J Hypertens 17:405–411, 1999

Harvey PJ, Molloy D, Upton J, et al: Dose response effect of conjugated equine oestrogen on blood pressure in postmenopausal women with hypertension. Blood Press 9:275–282, 2000

Hays J, Ockene JK, Brunner RL, et al: Effects of estrogen plus progestin on health-related quality of life. N Engl J Med 348:1839–1854, 2003

Hayward CS, Samaras K, Campbell L, et al: Effect of combination hormone replacement therapy on ambulatory blood pressure and arterial stiffness in diabetic postmenopausal women. Am J Hypertens 14:699–703, 2001

Herrington DM, Reboussin DM, Brosnihan KB, et al: Effects of estrogen replacement on the progression of coronary-artery atherosclerosis. N Engl J Med 343:522–529, 2000

Herrington DM, Espeland MA, Crouse JR 3rd, et al: Estrogen replacement and brachial artery flow-mediated vasodilation in older women. Arterioscler Thromb Vasc Biol 21:1955–1961, 2001

Herrington DM, Howard TD, Brosnihan KB, et al: Common estrogen receptor polymorphism augments effects of hormone replacement therapy on E-selectin but not C-reactive protein. Circulation 105:1879–1882, 2002

Hjerl K, Andersen EW, Keiding N, et al: Increased incidence of affective disorders, anxiety disorders, and non-natural mortality in women after breast cancer diagnosis: a nation-wide cohort study in Denmark. Acta Psychiatr Scand 105:258–264, 2002

Hjerl K, Andersen EW, Keiding N, et al: Depression as a prognostic factor for breast cancer mortality. Psychosomatics 44:24–30, 2003

Hochberg MC, Kasper J, Williamson J, et al: The contribution of osteoarthritis to disability: preliminary data from the Women's Health and Aging Study. J Rheumatol 22 (suppl 43):16–18, 1995

Horsten M, Mittleman MA, Wamala SP, et al: Depressive symptoms and lack of social integration in relation to prognosis of CHD in middle-aged women. The Stockholm Female Coronary Risk Study. Eur Heart J 21:1072–1080, 2000

House A, Knapp P, Bamford J, et al: Mortality at 12 and 24 months after stroke may be associated with depressive symptoms at 1 month. Stroke 32:696–701, 2001

Hulka BS, Chambless LE, Deubner DC, et al: Breast cancer and estrogen replacement therapy. Am J Obstet Gynecol 143:638–644, 1982

Hulley S, Grady D, Bush T, et al: Randomized trial of estrogen plus progestin for secondary prevention of coronary heart disease in postmenopausal women. Heart and Estrogen/progestin Replacement Study (HERS) Research Group. JAMA 280:605–613, 1998

Hux MJ, O'Brian BJ, Iskedjian M, et al: Relation between severity of Alzheimer's disease and costs of caring. CMAJ 159:457–465, 1998

Iwamoto J, Takeda T, Ichimura S: Forearm bone mineral density in postmenopausal women with rheumatoid arthritis. Calcif Tissue Int 70:1–8, 2002

Jiang YG, Chen JK, Wu ZL: Promotive effect of diethylstilbestrol on urethan-induced mouse lung tumorigenesis. Chemosphere 41:187–190, 2000

Johnson KA, Jones K, Holman BL, et al: Preclinical prediction of Alzheimer's disease using SPECT. Neurology 50:1563–1571, 1998

Jonas BS, Mussolino ME: Symptoms of depression as a prospective risk factor for stroke. Psychosom Med 62:463–471, 2000

Jorge RE, Robinson RG, Arndt S, et al: Mortality and poststroke depression: a placebo-controlled trial of antidepressants. Am J Psychiatry 160:1823–1829, 2003

Jorm AE, Jolley D: The incidence of dementia: a meta-analysis. Neurology 51:728–733, 1998

Kado DM, Browner WS, Palermo L, et al: Vertebral fractures and mortality in older women: a prospective study. Study of Osteoporotic Fractures Research Group. Arch Intern Med 159:1215–1220, 1999

Kanaya AM, Herrington D, Vittinghoff E, et al: Glycemic effects of postmenopausal hormone therapy: the Heart and Estrogen/progestin Replacement Study. Ann Intern Med 138:1–9, 2003

Kanik KS, Wilder RL: Hormonal alterations in rheumatoid arthritis, including the effects of pregnancy. Rheum Dis Clin North Am 26:805–823, 2000

Kanis JA, WHO Study Group: Assessment of fracture risk and its application to screening for postmenopausal osteoporosis: synopsis of a WHO report. Osteoporos Int 4:368–381, 1994

Kannel WB, Hjortland MC, McNamara PM, et al: Menopause and risk of cardiovascular disease: the Framingham Study. Ann Intern Med 85:447–452, 1976

Kawecka-Jaszcz K, Czarnecka D, Olszanecka A, et al: The effect of hormone replacement therapy on arterial blood pressure and vascular compliance in postmenopausal women with arterial hypertension. J Hum Hypertens 16:509–516, 2002

Kessler RC, Berglund P, Demler O, et al: The epidemiology of major depressive disorder: results from the National Comorbidity Survey Replication (NCS-R). JAMA 289:3095–3105, 2003

Khamashta MA, Ruiz-Irastorza G, Hughes GR: Systemic lupus erythematosus flares during pregnancy. Rheum Dis Clin North Am 23:15–30, 1997

Kiss E, Bhattoa HP, Bettembuk P, et al: Pregnancy in women with systemic lupus erythematosus. Eur J Obstet Gynecol Reprod Biol 101:129–134, 2002

Koepsell TD, Dugowson CE, Nelson JL, et al: Non-contraceptive hormones and the risk of rheumatoid arthritis in menopausal women. Int J Epidemiol 23:1248–1255, 1994

Kotila M, Numminen H, Waltimo O, et al: Depression after stroke: results of the FINNSTROKE Study. Stroke 29:368–372, 1998

Koutsavlis AT, Wolfson C: Elements of mobility as predictors of survival in elderly patients with dementia: findings from the Canadian Study of Health and Aging. Chronic Dis Can 21:93–103, 2000

Kroger H, Honkanen R, Saarikoski S, et al: Decreased axial bone mineral density in perimenopausal women with rheumatoid arthritis: a population-based study. Ann Rheum Dis 53:18–23, 1994

Lacey JV Jr, Mink PJ, Lubin JH, et al: Menopausal hormone replacement therapy and risk of ovarian cancer. JAMA 288:334–341, 2002

Lauritzen JB, Petersen MM, Lund B: Effect of external hip protectors on hip fractures. Lancet 341:11–13, 1993

LeBlanc ES, Janowsky J, Chan BK, et al: Hormone replacement therapy and cognition: systematic review and meta-analysis. JAMA 285:1489–1499, 2001

Leech JA, Dulberg C, Kellie S, et al: Relationship of lung function to severity of osteoporosis in women. Am Rev Respir Dis 141:68–71, 1990

Liao ML, Wang JH, Wang HM, et al: A study of the association between squamous cell carcinoma and adenocarcinoma in the lung, and history of menstruation in Shanghai women, China. Lung Cancer 14 (suppl 1):S215–S221, 1996

Lodder MC, Haugeberg G, Lems WF, et al: Radiographic damage associated with low bone mineral density and vertebral deformities in rheumatoid arthritis: the Oslo-Truro-Amsterdam (OSTRA) Collaborative Study. Arthritis Rheum 49:209–215, 2003

Looker AC, Orwoll ES, Johnston CC Jr, et al: Prevalence of low femoral neck bone density in older U.S. adults from NHANES III. J Bone Miner Res 12:1761–1768, 1997

MacDonald AG, Murphy EA, Capell HA, et al: Effects of hormone replacement therapy in rheumatoid arthritis: a double blind placebo-controlled study. Ann Rheum Dis 53:54–57, 1994

Manson JE, Hsia J, Johnson KC, et al: Estrogen plus progestin and the risk of coronary heart disease. Women's Health Initiative Investigators. N Engl J Med 349:523–534, 2003

Manwaring P, Morfis L, Diamond T, et al: Effects of hormone replacement therapy on ambulatory blood pressure and vascular responses in normotensive women: randomized controlled trial. Blood Press 9:22–27, 2000

Massie MK, Popkin MK: Depressive disorders, in Psycho-oncology. Edited by Holland JC. New York, Oxford University Press, 1998, pp 518–540

McBee WL, Dailey ME, Dugan E, et al: Hormone replacement therapy and other potential treatments for dementias. Endocrinol Metab Clin North Am 26:329–345, 1997

Medical Research Council: MRC stops study of long term use of HRT. Press release 23 October 2002. Available at: http://www.mrc.ac.uk/prn/index/public-interest/public-press_office/public-press_releases_2002/public-23_october_2002.htm. Accessed December 15, 2003.

Melton LJ 3rd, Chrischilles EA, Cooper C, et al: Perspective: how many women have osteoporosis? J Bone Miner Res 7:1005–1010, 1992

Mendelsohn ME: Mechanisms of estrogen action in the cardiovascular system. J Steroid Biochem Mol Biol 74:337–343, 2000

Mendelsohn ME: Protective effects of estrogen on the cardiovascular system. Am J Cardiol 89:12E–18E, 2002

Meyer WR, Costello N, Straneva P, et al: Effect of low-dose estrogen on hemodynamic response to stress: randomized controlled trial. Fertil Steril 75:394–399, 2001

Miller J, Chan BKS, Nelson HD: Postmenopausal estrogen replacement and risk for venous thromboembolism: a systematic review and meta-analysis for the U.S. Preventive Services Task Force. Ann Intern Med 136:680–690, 2002

Million Women Study Collaborators: Breast cancer and hormone-replacement therapy in the Million Women Study. Lancet 362:419–427, 2003

Mosca L, Manson JE, Sutherland SE, et al: Cardiovascular disease in women: a statement for healthcare professionals from the American Heart Association. Circulation 96:2468–2482, 1997

Mosca L, Collins P, Herrington DM, et al: Hormone replacement therapy and cardiovascular disease: a statement for healthcare professionals from the American Heart Association. Circulation 104:499–503, 2001

Nanda K, Bastian LA, Hasselblad V, et al: Hormone replacement therapy and the risk of colorectal cancer: a meta-analysis. Obstet Gynecol 93:880–888, 1999

National Osteoporosis Foundation: Osteoporosis: disease statistics, February 2004. Available at: http://www.nof.org/osteoporosis/stats.htm. Accessed March 30, 2004.

Neele SJ, Evertz R, De Valk-De Roo G: Effect of 1 year of discontinuation of raloxifene or estrogen therapy on bone mineral density after 5 years of treatment in healthy postmenopausal women. Bone 30:599–603, 2002

Nelson HD, Humphrey LL, Nygren P, et al: Postmenopausal hormone replacement therapy: scientific review. JAMA 288:872–881, 2002

Nevitt MC, Felson DT: Sex hormones and the risk of osteoarthritis in women: epidemiological evidence. Ann Rheum Dis 55:673–676, 1996

Nevitt MC, Thompson DE, Black DM, et al: Effect of alendronate on limited-activity days and bed-disability days caused by back pain in postmenopausal women with existing vertebral fractures. Fracture Intervention Trial Research Group. Arch Intern Med 160:77–85, 2000

Nevitt MC, Felson DT, Williams EN, et al: The effect of estrogen plus progestin on knee symptoms and related disability in postmenopausal women: the Heart and Estrogen/progestin Replacement Study, a randomized, double-blind, placebo-controlled trial. Arthritis Rheum 44:811–818, 2001

North American Menopause Society: Amended report from the NAMS Advisory Panel on Postmenopausal Hormone Therapy. Menopause 10:6–12, 2003

Ohira T, Iso H, Satoh S, et al: Prospective study of depressive symptoms and risk of stroke among Japanese. Stroke 32:903–908, 2001

Ostbye T, Hill G, Steenhuis R: Mortality in elderly Canadians with and without dementia: a five-year follow-up. Neurology 53:521–526, 1999

Ostensen M: Sex hormones and pregnancy in rheumatoid arthritis and systemic lupus erythematosus. Ann N Y Acad Sci 876:131–144, 1999

Osteoporosis prevention, diagnosis, and therapy. NIH Consens Statement 17:1–45, 2000

Ostir GV, Markides KS, Peek MK, et al: The association between emotional well-being and the incidence of stroke in older adults. Psychosom Med 63:210–215, 2001

Persson I, Weiderpass E, Bergkvist L, et al: Risks of breast and endometrial cancer after estrogen and estrogen-progestin replacement. Cancer Causes Control 10:253–260, 1999

Petersen RC, Smith GE, Waring SC, et al: Mild cognitive impairment: clinical characterization and outcome. Arch Neurol 56:303–308, 1999

Popovich JM, Fox PG, Burns KR: The impact of depression on stroke recovery in the U.S. Int J Psychiatr Nurs Res 7:842–855, 2002

Ramasubbu R, Patten SB: Effect of depression on stroke morbidity and mortality. Can J Psychiatry 48:250–257, 2003

Rapp SR, Espeland MA, Shumaker SA, et al: Effect of estrogen plus progestin on global cognitive function in postmenopausal women: the Women's Health Initiative Memory Study: a randomized controlled trial. WHIMS Investigators. JAMA 289:2663–2672, 2003

Reginster J[Y], Minne HW, Sorensen OH, et al: Randomized trial of the effects of risedronate on vertebral fractures in women with established postmenopausal osteoporosis: Vertebral Efficacy With Risedronate Therapy (VERT) Study Group. Osteoporos Int 11:83–91, 2000

Reginster JY, Kvasz A, Bruyere O, et al: Is there any rationale for prescribing hormone replacement therapy (HRT) to prevent or to treat osteoarthritis? Osteoarthritis Cartilage 11:87–91, 2003

Reynolds DL, Chambers LW, Badley EM, et al: Physical disability among Canadians reporting musculoskeletal diseases. J Rheumatol 19:1020–1030, 1992

Richette P, Corvol M, Bardin T: Estrogens, cartilage, and osteoarthritis. Joint Bone Spine 70:257–262, 2003

Rigler SK: Management of poststroke depression in older people. Clin Geriatr Med 15:765–783, 1999

Risch HA, Howe GR, Jain M, et al: Are female smokers at higher risk for lung cancer than male smokers? A case-control analysis by histologic type. Am J Epidemiol 138:281–293, 1993

Robinson RG: Poststroke depression: prevalence, diagnosis, treatment, and disease progression. Biol Psychiatry 54:376–387, 2003

Rockwood K, Stadnyk K: The prevalence of dementia in the elderly: a review. Can J Psychiatry 39:253–257, 1994

Saitta A, Altavilla D, Cucinotta D, et al: Randomized, double-blind, placebo-controlled study on effects of raloxifene and hormone replacement therapy on plasma NO concentrations, endothelin-1 levels, and endothelium-dependent vasodilation in postmenopausal women. Arterioscler Thromb Vasc Biol 21:1512–1519, 2001

Samaan SA, Crawford MH: Estrogen and cardiovascular function after menopause. J Am Coll Cardiol 26:1403–1410, 1995

Schairer C, Lubin J, Troisi R, et al: Menopausal estrogen and estrogen-progestin replacement therapy and breast cancer risk. JAMA 283:485–491, 2000

Scuteri A, Bos AJ, Brant LJ, et al: Hormone replacement therapy and longitudinal changes in blood pressure in postmenopausal women. Ann Intern Med 135:229–238, 2001a

Scuteri A, Lakatta EG, Bos AJ, et al: Effect of estrogen and progestin replacement on arterial stiffness indices in postmenopausal women. Aging (Milano) 13:122–130, 2001b

Schindler AE: Thyroid function and postmenopause. Gynecol Endocrinol 17:79–85, 2003

Sharpe M, Hawton K, House A, et al: Mood disorders in long-term survivors of stroke: associations with brain lesion location and volume. Psychol Med 20:815–828, 1990

Shenstone BD, Mahmoud A, Woodward R: Longitudinal bone mineral density changes in early rheumatoid arthritis. Br J Rheumatol 33:541–545, 1994

Shibuya K, Hagino H, Morio Y, et al: Cross-sectional and longitudinal study of osteoporosis in patients with rheumatoid arthritis. Clin Rheumatol 21:150–158, 2002

Shumaker SA, Legault C, Rapp SR, et al: Estrogen plus progestin and the incidence of dementia and mild cognitive impairment in postmenopausal women: the Women's Health Initiative Memory Study: a randomized controlled trial. WHIMS Investigators. JAMA 289:2651–2662, 2003

Shumaker SA, Legault C, Kuller L, et al: Conjugated equine estrogens and incidences of probable dementia and mild cognitive impairment in postmenopausal women: Women's Health Initiative Memory Study. JAMA 291:2947–2958, 2004

Siegfried JM: Women and lung cancer: does oestrogen play a role? Lancet Oncol 2:506–513, 2001

Sillero-Arenas M, Delgado RC, Rodriguez M, et al: Menopausal hormone replacement therapy and breast cancer: a meta-analysis. Obstet Gynecol 79:286–294, 1992

Simmonds P: Managing patients with lung cancer: new guidelines should improve standards of care. BMJ 319:527–528, 1999

Smith MY, Redd WH, Peyser C, et al: Post-traumatic stress disorder in cancer: a review. Psychooncology 8:521–537, 1999

Spector TD, Nandra D, Hart DJ, et al: Is hormone replacement therapy protective for hand and knee osteoarthritis in women? the Chingford Study. Ann Rheum Dis 56:432–434, 1997

Stabile LP, Siegfried JM: Sex and gender differences in lung cancer. J Gend Specif Med 6:37–48, 2003

Stabile LP, Gaither Davis AL, Gubish CT, et al: Human non–small cell lung tumors and cells derived from normal lung express both estrogen receptor alpha and beta and show biological responses to estrogen. Cancer Res 62:2141–2150, 2002

Stampfer MJ, Colditz GA, Willett WC, et al: Postmenopausal estrogen therapy and cardiovascular disease. Ten-year follow-up from the Nurses' Health Study. N Engl J Med 325:756–762, 1991

Steinberg KK, Thacker SB, Smith SJ, et al: A meta-analysis of the effect of estrogen replacement therapy on the risk of breast cancer. JAMA 265:1985–1990, 1991

Sung BH, Ching M, Izzo JL Jr, et al: Estrogen improves abnormal norepinephrine-induced vasoconstriction in postmenopausal women. J Hypertens 17:523–528, 1999

Swenson JR, O'Connor CM, Barton D, et al: Influence of depression and effect of treatment with sertraline on quality of life after hospitalization for acute coronary syndrome. Sertraline Antidepressant Heart Attack Randomized Trial (SADHART) Group. Am J Cardiol 92:1271–1276, 2003

Taioli E, Wynder EL: Re: endocrine factors and adenocarcinoma of the lung in women. J Natl Cancer Inst 86:869–870, 1994

Todaro JF, Shen BJ, Niaura R, et al: Effect of negative emotions on frequency of coronary heart disease (the Normative Aging Study). Am J Cardiol 92:901–906, 2003

Torgerson DJ, Bell-Syer SE: Hormone replacement therapy and prevention of nonvertebral fractures: a meta-analysis of randomized trials. JAMA 285:2891–2897, 2001

Tremollieres FA, Pouilles JM, Ribot C: Withdrawal of hormone replacement therapy is associated with significant vertebral bone loss in postmenopausal women. Osteoporos Int 12:385–390, 2001

Tsai CL, Liu TK: Osteoarthritis in women: its relationship to estrogen and current trends. Life Sci 50:1737–1744, 1992

Ushiyama T, Ueyama H, Inoue K, et al: Estrogen receptor gene polymorphism and generalized osteoarthritis. J Rheumatol 25:134–137, 1998

U.S. Food and Drug Administration: FDA approves new labeling and provides new advice to postmenopausal women who use or who are considering using estrogen and estrogen with progestin. FDA Fact Sheet, January 8, 2003. Available at: http://www.fda.gov/bbs/topics/factsheets/2003/fsl.html. Accessed December 15, 2003.

U.S. Preventive Services Task Force: Guide to Clinical Preventive Services, 2nd Edition. 1996. Available at: http://www.ncbi.nlm.nih.gov/books/bv.fcgi?rid=hstat3.chapter.10062. Accessed November 3, 2004.

U.S. Preventive Services Task Force: Guide to Clinical Preventive Services, 3rd Edition. Recommendations. 2000. Available at: http://www.ncbi.nlm.nih.gov/books/bv.fcgi?rid=hstat3.part.1. Accessed November 3, 2004.

U.S. Preventive Services Task Force: Postmenopausal hormone replacement therapy for the primary prevention of chronic conditions: recommendations and rationale. Ann Intern Med 137:834–839, 2002

van den Brink HR, van Everdingen AA, van Wijk MJ: Adjuvant oestrogen therapy does not improve disease activity in postmenopausal patients with rheumatoid arthritis. Ann Rheum Dis 52:862–865, 1993

Viscoli CM, Brass LM, Kernan WN, et al: A clinical trial of estrogen-replacement therapy after ischemic stroke. N Engl J Med 345:1243–1249, 2001

Vongpatanasin W, Tuncel M, Mansour Y, et al: Transdermal estrogen replacement therapy decreases sympathetic activity in postmenopausal women. Circulation 103:2903–2908, 2001

Walsh BW, Kuller LH, Wild RA, et al: Effects of raloxifene on serum lipids and coagulation factors in healthy postmenopausal women. JAMA 279:1445–1451, 1998

Walsh BW, Paul S, Wild RA, et al: The effects of hormone replacement therapy and raloxifene on C-reactive protein and homocysteine in healthy postmenopausal women: a randomized, controlled trial. J Clin Endocrinol Metab 85:214–218, 2000

Walsh BW, Cox DA, Sashegyi A, et al: Role of tumor necrosis factor-alpha and inter-leukin-6 in the effects of hormone replacement therapy and raloxifene on C-reactive protein in postmenopausal women. Am J Cardiol 88:825–828, 2001

Wassertheil-Smoller S, Hendrix SL, Limacher M, et al: Effect of estrogen plus progestin on stroke in postmenopausal women: the Women's Health Initiative: a randomized trial. JAMA 289:2673–2684, 2003

Wathen CN, Feig DS, Feightner JS, et al: Hormone replacement therapy for the primary prevention of chronic disease: recommendation statement from the Canadian Task Force on Preventive Health Care. CMAJ 170:1535–1537, 2004

Wiart L, Petit H, Joseph PA: Fluoxetine in early poststroke depression: a double-blind placebo-controlled study. Stroke 31:1829–1832, 2000

Wiktorowicz ME, Goeree R, Papaioannou A, et al: Economic implications of hip fracture: health service use, institutional care and cost in Canada. Osteoporos Int 12:271–278, 2001

Wilkinson PR, Wolfe CD, Warburton FG, et al: A long-term follow-up of stroke patients. Stroke 28:507–512, 1997

Williams JI, Iron K, Wu K: Estimating the impact of arthritis on the burden of disability and the costs of health services, in Patterns of Health Care in Ontario: Arthritis and Related Conditions. Edited by Williams JI, Badley EM. Toronto, ON, Institute for Clinical Evaluative Sciences, 1998, pp 11–26

Wilson PW, Garrison RJ, Castelli WP: Postmenopausal estrogen use, cigarette smoking, and cardiovascular morbidity in women over 50: the Framingham Study. N Engl J Med 313:1038–1043, 1985

Wluka AE, Cicuttini FM, Spector TD: Menopause, oestrogens and arthritis. Maturitas 35:183–199, 2000

Wluka AE, Davis SR, Bailey M, et al: Users of oestrogen replacement therapy have more knee cartilage than non-users. Ann Rheum Dis 60:332–336, 2001

Wolf H, Grunwald M, Ecke GM, et al: The prognosis of mild cognitive impairment in the elderly. J Neural Transm 54:31–50, 1998

Women's Health Initiative Steering Committee: Effects of conjugated equine estrogen in postmenopausal women with hysterectomy: the Women's Health Initiative randomized controlled trial. JAMA 291:1701–1712, 2004

Women's Health Initiative Study Group: Design of the Women's Health Initiative clinical trial and observational study. Control Clin Trials 19:61–109, 1998

Writing Group for the PEPI Trial: Effects of estrogen or estrogen/progestin regimens on heart disease risk factors in postmenopausal women: the Postmenopausal Estrogen/Progestin Interventions (PEPI) Trial. JAMA 273:199–208, 1995

Writing Group for the Women's Health Initiative Investigators: Risks and benefits of estrogen plus progestin in healthy postmenopausal women. JAMA 288:321–333, 2002

Wulsin LR, Singal BM: Do depressive symptoms increase the risk for the onset of coronary disease? A systematic quantitative review. Psychosom Med 65:201–210, 2003

Wyss JM, Carlson SH: Effects of hormone replacement therapy on the sympathetic nervous system and blood pressure. Curr Hypertens Rep 5:241–246, 2003

Yaffe K, Sawaya G, Lieberburg I, et al: Estrogen therapy in postmenopausal women: effects on cognitive function and dementia. JAMA 279:688–695, 1998

Zang EA, Wynder EL: Differences in lung cancer risk between men and women: examination of the evidence. J Natl Cancer Inst 88:183–192, 1996

Zweifel JE, O'Brien WH: A meta-analysis of the effect of hormone replacement therapy upon depressed mood. Psychoneuroendocrinology 22:189–212 [erratum, 22:655], 1997

Chapter 7

Gynecologic Aspects of Perimenopause and Menopause

Diana L. Dell, M.D., F.A.C.O.G.

*M*enopause is the medical term that, strictly defined, means that a woman has not had menstrual bleeding for a full year (Utian 2001). See the preface to this volume for definitions of *menopause* and related terms. In this chapter, I will review the changes and symptoms associated with the menopausal transition and beyond and discuss their gynecologic management. The average age for cessation of menses in North American and northern European women is 51 years. Perimenopausal symptoms are described between ages 45 and 55 years and usually last 4–5 years. A woman experiencing natural cessation of menses prior to age 40 has *premature menopause,* and a woman experiencing natural cessation of menses after age 55 has *late menopause. Surgical menopause* occurs when both ovaries are removed before natural menopause has occurred.

The transition through menopause is a multifactorial process involving decreased ovarian function, sociocultural factors, and individual psychological factors that act individually or in concert to produce perimenopausal symptoms (Sherwin 2001).

Physiology of Perimenopause

A fuller description of the physiology of perimenopause and menopause can be found in Chapter 3, Effects of Reproductive Hormones and Selective Estrogen Receptor Modulators on the Central Nervous System During Menopause. The physiologic responsibility of a human ovary is both reproductive (periodic release of oocytes plus steroid hormones to sustain reproductive function) and endocrinological (nonreproductive effects of estrogen, progesterone, and testosterone on bone, mood, etc.).

In utero, after ovarian development has occurred, there is active follicular activity in the fetal ovary, presumably in response to transplacental maternal hormone. Until recently, we believed that when a female was born, she had all the oocytes she would ever possess residing in her ovaries in an arrested prophase of meiosis. Newer data indicate that later oogenesis can occur in some circumstances. In childhood, with an absence of gonadal hormones, the ovary becomes dormant until puberty. Pubertal changes are orchestrated by complex changes in the hypothalamic-pituitary-adrenal axis that initiate progressive responsiveness from the oocyte and follicle, which creates reproductive capacity. For the next 30–40 years, estrogen production and follicular maturation sustain adult reproductive capacity via repeated monthly ovulations. At this level of estrogen production, the nonreproductive estrogen-dependent systems are also sustained. With the aging of the ovary, there is a marked decrease in both the number of remaining follicular units and their sensitivity to gonadotropin (follicle-stimulating hormone [FSH], luteinizing hormone [LH], inhibin) stimulation. Over time, cyclic changes result in fewer successful ovulations and less estrogen is produced, in spite of increasing FSH and LH production. Eventually, so little estrogen is produced that endometrial proliferation cannot be maintained, and menopause ensues (Speroff et al. 1999).

The progression through perimenopause to menopause ranges over a period of years. In the later stages of this transition, women may experience menstrual bleeding even though their estradiol levels are low and their FSH is in the postmenopausal range (FSH > 40 mIU/mL); typically, LH will remain in the normal range during this interval. Eventually, elevated levels of both FSH and LH provide conclusive clinical evidence of ovarian senescence or failure (Byyny and Speroff 1996).

After natural menopause, testosterone levels do not initially fall appreciably—probably because elevated LH drives the remaining stromal tissue in the ovary to increase testosterone secretion. Over time, circulating levels of androstenedione fall to about half the premenopausal level, which is mostly of adrenal origin. Postmenopausally, estrone replaces estradiol as the dominant estrogen and the average estrone level is 30–70 pg/mL. Estrone is de-rived primarily from the peripheral conversion of androstenedione; the percentage of conversion of androstenedione to estrogen correlates with body weight—higher weight being associated with higher conversion. Cir-culating estradiol levels postmenopause are between 10 and 20 pg/mL, most of which is derived from the peripheral conversion of estrone (Speroff et al. 1999).

Symptoms Associated With Perimenopause and Menopause

In cultures where the menopausal transition has been medicalized into a "menopausal syndrome," numerous physical and psychological symptoms have been attributed to declining estrogen levels (Lock 1998). See Chapter 2, Physiology and Symptoms of Menopause, for further discussion of these symptoms.

In addition to symptoms that any perimenopausal woman may experi-ence, women with premature menopause may be surprised and especially distressed by the prospect of premature aging and early loss of fertility.

Changes in Menstrual Character

As women move through the menopausal transition, changes in menstrual function are common. Although a minority of women will just stop having menses, the majority will experience changes in their menstrual cycle over several years. Women in their mid-30s will often note that the menstrual cy-cle length becomes shorter (<28 days) and menstrual flow lasts for a shorter period than at earlier ages. When women approach the menopausal transi-tion, menses become irregular as ovulatory frequency declines. Late in peri-menopause, women may skip several periods and then start cyclic menstrual bleeding again for a few months.

Practitioners should not assume that all bleeding during this transition is benign. Evaluation by a gynecologist is indicated for extremely heavy bleeding, spotting between cycles, and bleeding with intercourse. Although the majority of these abnormalities will ultimately be attributable to anovu-latory cycles, endometrial biopsy or other diagnostic procedures may be needed to rule out more serious disorders (endometrial hyperplasia and cer-vical and endometrial cancer). See Table 7–1 for methods of investigating perimenopausal bleeding.

Symptoms caused by hormonal dysregulation are usually treated with low-dose oral contraceptives or hormone therapy. Nonmalignant conditions

TABLE 7–1.   Evaluation of perimenopausal bleeding

Method	Purpose
Pregnancy test	Rule out bleeding secondary to pregnancy/miscarriage
Cervical inspection	Rule out lesions on cervix as cause of bleeding
Pelvic examination	Rule out uterine enlargement or masses
	Rule out ovarian masses
Uterine ultrasound	Measure uterine lining (<3 mm thickness is normal)
Endometrial biopsy	Office procedure—aspiration or scraping of endometrial cells for cytological evaluation
Hysteroscopy	Office or surgical procedure—visualization of endometrial cavity with or without endometrial sampling
D and C (dilatation and curettage)	Surgical procedure—dilatation of the cervix to allow scraping of endometrial lining from uterine walls; for cytological examination

Note.   Management strategies are directed toward early detection of endometrial hyperplasia. Any bleeding between menstrual cycles or during intercourse should be evaluated.

associated with heavy bleeding include polyps in the cervical canal or uterine cavity, fibroid tumors that prevent normal endometrial development, and abnormal clotting function. These disorders may be treated by hysteroscopy, dilatation and curettage (D and C), endometrial ablation, or hysterectomy.

Vasomotor Symptoms

The Study of Women's Health Across the Nation (SWAN) investigated the relationships among multiple factors associated with menopause among women in the United States. The study included 12,425 women ages 40–55 years, the majority of whom were premenopausal or in early perimenopause. Community-based participants from seven regions across the United States were surveyed between 1995 and 1997. The majority of these women (12,357) reported hot flashes and night sweats. Vasomotor symptoms were reported most frequently among African American women (45.5%), Hispanic women (35.4%), and Caucasian women (31.2%). Women of Asian ancestry were much less likely to report vasomotor symptoms (Chinese women, 20.5%; Japanese women, 17.6%). Late perimenopausal women reported more symptoms than premenopausal women. Women who had experienced surgical menopause were more likely to report vasomotor symptoms than women who were naturally menopausal (Gold et al. 2000).

Higher body mass index, premenstrual symptoms, perceived stress, use of over-the-counter pain medications, and older age were also significantly associated with vasomotor symptoms. However, fewer women with postgraduate education reported experiencing vasomotor symptoms (Gold et al. 2004).

In another survey of 501 untreated women, 50% began experiencing hot flashes when their menstrual cycle was still regular or just becoming irregular. Most of the remaining women began having symptoms within 1 year of menopause, although a few began having symptoms within 2 years of menopause. Duration of vasomotor symptoms in the majority of women (60%) was less than 7 years, but 15% reported symptoms for more than 15 years (Kronenberg 1990).

It is also important to note that more than estrogen levels are operative with the vasomotor phenomenon. Psychosocial factors such as individual expectations, stressful contexts, and cultural norms appear to moderate the experience and reporting of hot flashes. For example, researchers conducting physiological monitoring during stressful and nonstressful laboratory conditions found that perimenopausal women who were having frequent hot flashes outside the laboratory had more objectively detectable hot flashes and subjective hot flashes under stressful conditions (Stanton et al. 2002). Hot flashes may also accompany some common medical conditions (e.g., thyroid disease, leukemia, carcinoid, pheochromocytoma) and common psychiatric conditions (e.g., anxiety disorders, panic symptoms, substance withdrawal).

Although the underlying mechanism for hot flashes is poorly understood, complex interactions occurring in both the central nervous system and peripherally are operative. Peripherally, there is a sudden onset of reddened skin over the head, neck, and chest; it is accompanied by a feeling of intense body heat and sometimes by profuse perspiration (Speroff et al. 1999). Centrally, LH surges and hypothalamic norepinephrine activity increases before the hot flash; β-endorphins decrease at the onset of a hot flash and rise significantly after it; after the hot flash, adrenocorticotropic hormone and growth hormone also rise (Ginsburg 1994).

The symptoms that accompany hot flashes (e.g., facial flushing, perspiration, and palpitations) contribute to the discomfort, inconvenience, and even embarrassment reported by women in some cultures. At the opposite end of the culture spectrum are women from Japanese, Chinese, and Mayan cultures, where there is not even a word to describe hot flashes (Speroff et al. 1999). Other factors such as diet, climate, genetics, and reproductive history undoubtedly play a role in the attribution of discomfort from hot flashes (Robinson 1996). Nonetheless, in Western cultures the majority of women who initiate hormone treatment are seeking relief from menopausal symptoms (48%), with osteoporosis prevention being the second most common reason (32%) (Newton et al. 1997).

Treatment of vasomotor symptoms is a U.S. Food and Drug Administration (FDA)–approved indication for estrogen or estrogen/progesterone therapy at the "lowest dose, and shortest time possible." The response to hormone therapy is generally rapid, with measurable improvement in both frequency and intensity of vasomotor symptoms occurring within 1–2 weeks; continued improvement is noted over time (Derman et al. 1995). See also Chapter 2, Physiology and Symptoms of Menopause.

Sleep Disturbances

As women progress through perimenopause, symptomatic individuals often present with complaints related to insomnia, irritability, and mood disturbances. Nighttime hot flashes tend to occur with the onset of rapid eye movement (REM) sleep, thus directly disturbing sleep architecture. Perimenopausal women also report difficulty falling asleep, difficulty maintaining sleep, and early morning awakening. Although numerous studies have shown insomnia symptoms to be estrogen dependent, the brain mechanism remains unclear, and circulating estrogen levels do not predict the intensity of subjective symptoms. Estrogen potentially has direct central effects on sleep regulatory areas of the hypothalamus and hippocampus.

A subjective improvement in sleep is commonly among the first changes women notice after initiating estrogen therapy. Experimentally, most studies show that estrogen improves sleep quality, even in the absence of vasomotor symptoms (Polo-Kantola et al. 1998). Estrogen decreases sleep latency (Scharf et al. 1997), decreases night sweats and waking disturbances (Erlik et al. 1981), and increases REM sleep (Schiff et al. 1980).

Large numbers of perimenopausal and menopausal women have sleep-related problems. One study showed that 80% of women between ages 45 and 65 years ($n=886$, 70% postmenopausal) were using some form of alternative therapy to improve sleep (e.g., massage, soy, herbals, or stress management; Newton et al. 2002). What is less clear is the role that estrogen deficiency plays in causing or perpetuating sleep disturbances in this age group—and what impact sleep changes may have on mood symptoms during this time.

Mood Changes

Chapter 3, Effects of Reproductive Hormones and Selective Estrogen Receptor Modulators on the Central Nervous System During Menopause, and Chapter 4, Mood Disorders, Midlife, and Reproductive Aging, provide a full discussion of depression, anxiety, and irritability during midlife transitions.

Cognitive Changes

Benign changes in cognition occur with aging, but many menopausal women complain of temporary cognitive changes (verbal memory) specifically associated with the menopausal transition. Because estrogen affects brain function in multiple ways—that is, estrogen increases cerebral blood flow, increases glucose transport, enhances neurite branching, enhances the effects of other neurotransmitters, and has neuroprotective effects (e.g., protecting neurons from oxidative stress, preventing glutamate toxicity)—loss of estrogen could be expected to affect cognition (Birge 2000). Experimentally, ovarian suppression has demonstrated declines in verbal memory in young women that were reversed when estrogen was added back (Sherwin and Tulandi 1996). In a study of postmenopausal women taking estrogen or placebo, functional magnetic resonance imaging detected increased activity in anterior frontal lobes and inferior parietal lobes (cognitive areas) of women using estrogen (Shaywitz et al. 1999). Further information about the effects of gonadal steroid hormones on the central nervous system can be found in Chapter 3, Effects of Reproductive Hormones and Selective Estrogen Receptor Modulators on the Central Nervous System During Menopause, and Chapter 6, Medical Aspects of Perimenopause and Menopause.

Sexual Dysfunction

Changes in sexual function associated with aging and menopause are very common. Avis and colleagues (2000) reported that about 40% of women ages 51–61 years ($n=200$) had lower sexual desire than they did when they were in their 40s. Additionally, 37% had difficulty reaching orgasm, and 23% had pain with intercourse. Other researchers have confirmed decreased sexual responsivity, decreased sexual frequency, lower libido, increased vaginal pain, and increased partner problems (Dennerstein et al. 2001).

Etiologies of these sexual changes are multifactorial: aging, aging of the partner, changes in general health, use of medications, and loss of gonadal hormones. Estradiol levels of less than 50 pg/mL have been associated with increased vaginal dryness, pain with penetration, pain with intercourse, and vaginal burning (Sarrel 2000).

Genital Changes

Decreasing estrogen levels ultimately cause the vaginal mucosa to be measurably thinner, dryer, and less elastic; vaginal secretions decrease (both baseline and in response to sexual stimulation); and vaginal pH increases. Although changes in the vaginal mucosa are often considered "late" changes associated with menopause, Dennerstein and associates (2001) demonstrated that 25% of women report vaginal dryness at 1 year after menopause, and 47% at 3 years after menopause. By 4 years postmenopause, vaginal atrophy can be documented in 60% of women not treated with estrogen (Versi et al. 2001). Estrogen therapy can rapidly reverse these changes and reduce dyspareunia (Willhite and O'Connell 2001), whether delivered vaginally, orally, or transcutaneously. Other therapies may also be helpful, especially lubricants and moisturizers that are available without prescription.

Changes in vulvar skin mirror the skin changes taking place in other areas of the body: increased dryness, decreased collagen content, decreased skin thickness, decreased elasticity, impaired wound healing, and increased susceptibility to infection. Skin changes can be documented early in postmenopause and respond to estrogen therapy (Brincat et al. 1987). See also Chapter 2, Physiology and Symptoms of Menopause.

Urinary Incontinence

Urinary symptoms can also occur as estrogen levels decrease. There is thinning of the urethral lining and shortening of the urethra. Relaxation of the muscles of the pelvic floor may also distort the anatomical position of the bladder neck. These changes often lead to incontinence (persistent involuntary leakage of urine) and recurrent urinary tract infections. Current estimates are that about 30% of women experience urinary incontinence, although less than half of these women seek medical help for the condition (Grodstein et al. 2003).

Urinary incontinence and recurrent urinary tract infections should not be considered inevitable consequences of aging. At least 50% of women with urinary stress incontinence (involuntary loss of urine associated with lifting, laughing, coughing, or sneezing) will improve with Kegel exercises (Kegel exercises consist of practicing the voluntary contraction of the perineal muscles that control the flow of urine). Anticholinergics and smooth muscle relaxants are also used to alter bladder contractions, which improves urge incontinence (loss of urine associated with feeling the need to urinate but being unable to get to a toilet in time). New compounds such as duloxetine are currently showing promising results in clinical trials.

Women with either type of urinary incontinence should be referred for evaluation by a urogynecologist or urologist. While awaiting evaluation, the patient should receive a urinalysis to rule out infection and should be treated with antibiotics if results are positive. Many women try to restrict fluid intake to prevent urine loss, but that may actually predispose them to more incontinence and a greater risk of infection. While awaiting evaluation, she can also begin Kegel exercises and avoid bladder irritants like alcohol, tobacco, and acidic foods.

Changes in Bone Density

One of the most significant (albeit silent) changes associated with menopausal estrogen deficiency is an acceleration of bone loss. For a full discussion of bone density and osteoporosis, see Chapter 6, Medical Aspects of Perimenopause and Menopause.

Cardiovascular Changes

Another change that begins rather silently in the postmenopause is an increasing risk of cardiovascular disease, which includes coronary heart disease, congestive heart disease, peripheral vascular disease, and stroke. For a full discussion of these conditions, see Chapter 6, Medical Aspects of Perimenopause and Menopause.

Women's Health Initiative

The Women's Health Initiative (WHI) is an ongoing National Institutes of Health–sponsored, randomized, multicenter trial designed to assess the long-term risks and benefits of conjugated equine estrogen (CEE; trade name, Premarin) and the combination CEE+MPA (medroxyprogesterone acetate; trade name, Provera) in chronic disease prevention. It planned to enroll 27,000 women ages 50–79 years, and the trial was originally scheduled to conclude in 2005 but was terminated early by the data safety monitoring board (Women's Health Initiative Study Group 1998; Writing Group for the Women's Health Initiative Investigators 2002). See Chapter 6, Medical Aspects of Perimenopause and Menopause, for details on the WHI.

A separate portion of the WHI, the Women's Health Initiative Memory Study (WHIMS), began in May 1996. This randomized, double-blind, placebo-controlled trial enrolled postmenopausal women older than 65 years who were participants in the WHI (receiving CEE+MPA or placebo). The primary outcome measure was "probable dementia," and the secondary outcome was "mild cognitive impairment" as identified by structured clinical assessment. See Chapter 6, Medical Aspects of Perimenopause and Menopause, for details on WHIMS.

Much of the difficulty in understanding the WHI and WHIMS results comes from how discordant these results are from 30 years of observational studies that preceded the trials. Grimes and Lobo (2002) identified four areas of bias that were built into the observational studies that account for those differences: selection bias, adherence bias, surveillance bias, and survivor bias. First, women choosing to receive hormone therapy in the observational studies were healthier users; they were younger, leaner, more likely to use moderate alcohol (protective effect), more physically active, and less likely to have a worrisome family history, smoke cigarettes, or have diabetes. Second, they were more adherent to their prescribed regimens (adherence is a marker for person characteristics associated with better health). Third, these women were seen more often by their physicians to receive prescriptions and benefited from better screening. And finally, some shrinking of the population occurs when women die of other diseases, leaving a healthier observation pool. These inherent biases of observational research often foster favorable conclusions (Grimes and Lobo 2002).

Who Should Take Hormones?

See Table 7–2 for efficacy and levels of evidence for estrogen use for various conditions. The short-term use of hormone therapy for relief of severe menopausal symptoms is likely to have more benefit than risk in appropriately screened patients. None of the prospective trials (WHI or WHIMS) addressed the risks or benefits of women in this group (symptomatic women). Estrogen is approved by the FDA for relief of vasomotor symptoms and treatment of atrophic vaginitis but is no longer recommended for the prevention of chronic disease. Hormone therapies are commonly prescribed off-label for perimenopausal mood changes, cognitive changes, and decreased libido, and as adjunctive therapy in psychiatric illness (e.g., depression, anxiety, psychosis). Hormone therapy is absolutely contraindicated in the presence of estrogen-sensitive cancer, although some breast and endometrial cancer survivors elect to use estrogen under some circumstances (Byyny and Speroff 1996). It is also contraindicated in women with a history of venous thrombosis or embolism during pregnancy or while using hormones (birth control pills, hormone therapy), because of significant risk of recurrences.

Treatment Strategies for Depressed Perimenopausal Women

Initiation of therapy for perimenopausal women with depressive symptoms should be based on both personal history and the severity of illness. Estrogen therapy is an appropriate first-line treatment for women with mild depressive symptoms, prominent menopausal symptoms, and minimal past history. If improvement in menopausal symptoms does not improve depressive symptoms as well, an antidepressant and psychotherapy should be added.

TABLE 7–2.   Estrogen: efficacy and level of evidence

Indication	Observational data	Prospective data, evidence level[a]	FDA approved[b]
Hot flashes, night sweats	Yes	Yes, A	Yes
Sleep disturbances	Yes	Yes, B	No
Vaginal dryness	Yes	Yes, A	Yes
Bleeding—anovulatory	Yes	Yes, B	No
Bleeding—hyperplasia	No, makes worse	Worsens, B	No
Mood changes	Probably works	Mixed, B	No
Primary cognitive protection	May help	Mixed, B	No
Secondary cognitive protection	May help	Worsens, A	No
Sexual dysfunction— libido	May help	Mixed, B	No
Sexual dysfunction— anorgasmia	May help	Mixed, C	No
Sexual dysfunction—pain, atrophy	Yes	Yes, B	No
Urinary incontinence	May help	No, A	No

Note.   See Chapter 6, Medical Aspects of Perimenopause and Menopause, for efficacy for the medical conditions osteoporosis, cardiovascular disease, and colon cancer. FDA=U.S. Food and Drug Administration.

[a]*Evidence level A:* Large, high-quality, randomized, double-blind, placebo-controlled trials, meta-analysis.
Evidence level B: Lesser-quality randomized trials, retrospective studies, systematic reviews.
Evidence level C: Expert opinion, case series, uncontrolled studies, consensus statements.
[b]Estrogen use is FDA approved *at the lowest effective dose for the shortest time possible.* Dose and duration of use are determined clinically.

For women with moderate or severe symptoms of depression, regardless of previous history, treatment with an antidepressant should be initiated. Several case reports indicated efficacy for selective serotonin reuptake inhibitors in relieving hot flashes, and that effect has now been documented for both venlafaxine and paroxetine in randomized controlled trials (Loprinzi et al. 2001; Stearns et al. 2003). The mechanism of this proposed effect has not been elucidated, and clinically the effect is far less robust than treatment with estrogen. See Chapter 4, Mood Disorders, Midlife, and Reproductive Aging, for further information on menopause and mood.

In perimenopausal or postmenopausal women with treatment-resistant psychiatric disorders, augmentation therapy with estrogen has been used with mixed results. A role for estrogen augmentation in psychotic disorders in perimenopausal or postmenopausal women is also under investigation in multiple settings. More detailed information can be found in Chapter 5, Psychotic Illness in Women at Perimenopause and Menopause.

Estrogens

The most commonly prescribed estrogen is conjugated equine estrogen (CEE), which was the agent used in all the prospective studies. There is no evidence to presume or deny that other estrogen products would behave in a similar manner over time. The standard dose of CEE (Premarin) is 0.625 mg; equivalence in other preparations varies (e.g., estradiol 0.5 mg; estropipate 0.5 mg; ethinyl estradiol 0.02 mg). Recent interest in lowering estrogen doses has spawned new research to determine the effectiveness of lower doses for both menopausal symptom control and osteoporosis prevention. Women with surgical menopause often require higher estrogen doses in the initial phases of treatment. See Table 7–3 for commonly used estrogen preparations.

Oral estrogens are used more commonly than other forms. The oral route maximizes beneficial effects on cholesterol metabolism. Clinical experience suggests that women who develop depression, irritability, anxiety, or headaches while on CEE may still tolerate other forms of estrogen without these effects. Perimenopausal women who still need contraception and who tolerate combination oral contraceptives are good candidates for using low-dose birth control pills, if there are no other contraindications.

Transdermal estrogen preparations are the preferred route of administration for perimenopausal women with migraine headaches and women with liver disease. Vaginal preparations are often recommended when a more intense local effect is desired; about half of the vaginal dose will be reflected in subsequent systemic estrogen levels.

Progestins

Estrogen plus progesterone is recommended for perimenopausal women who still have their uterus, because unopposed estrogen increases the risk of endometrial cancer. Adding a progestin appears to dampen mood in a dose-dependent manner (Sherwin 1991). Despite ongoing debate about whether micronized progesterone causes fewer mood symptoms than MPA, both can cause similar symptoms in equivalent doses. Some clinicians have elected to use progesterone-containing intrauterine devices for women desiring estro-

TABLE 7–3. Commonly used estrogen preparations

Generic name	Brand names (U.S. or Canada)	Usual dose range	Route
Conjugated equine estrogen (CEE)	Premarin, CES, Congest	0.3–1.25 mg daily	Oral
Conjugated estrogen, synthetic	Cenestin	0.3–1.25 mg daily	Oral
Esterified estrogen	Menest	0.3–1.25 mg daily	Oral
Estradiol	Estrace, Estradiol	0.5–2 mg daily	Oral
	Gynodiol	1–5 mg monthly	IM
	Depo-Estradiol, Delestrogen	10–20 mg monthly	IM
Estradiol acetate vaginal ring	Femring	0.05–0.1 mg daily (replaced in vagina every 3 months)	Vaginal
Estradiol vaginal ring	Estring	2 mg daily (replaced in vagina every 3 months)	Vaginal
Estradiol transdermal	Alora, Climara, Esclim, Estraderm, FemPatch, Vivelle, Estradot, Oesclim	0.025–0.1 mg once or twice weekly	Patch
Estrogen cream	Premarin, Estrace	0.5–4 mg daily	Vaginal
Estrone	Estrone 5, EstraGyn 5	0.1–1 mg weekly	IM
Estropipate	Ogen, Ortho-Est	0.625–2.5 mg daily	Oral

Note. All listed preparations are used with progestin if the uterus is intact. IM=intramuscular.

TABLE 7–4.   Commonly used progestins in hormone therapy regimens

Generic name	Brand names (U.S. or Canada)	Usual dose range	Route
Medroxyprogesterone (MPA)	Provera, Amen	2.5–5 mg daily *or*	Oral
		5–10 mg daily for 12 days monthly	Oral
	Depo-Provera	150 mg every 3 months	IM
Norethindrone	Aygestin	2.5–5 mg daily *or*	Oral
		5–10 mg daily for 12 days monthly	Oral
Progesterone, micronized	Prometrium	100 mg daily *or*	Oral
		200 mg daily for 12 days monthly	Oral

Note.   IM=intramuscular.

gen therapy who cannot tolerate progestin side effects. Table 7–4 lists commonly used progestins.

Estrogen and progesterone can be used continuously or in a cyclic fashion. Cyclic regimens cause scheduled bleeding and may precipitate premenstrual syndrome–like symptoms. Continuous regimens often cause irregular spotting, which generally resolves within 1 year but is associated with patient dissatisfaction and discontinuation of therapy.

Combination Therapies

The combination of oral CEE+MPA has been in common use since 1994. See Table 7–5 for commonly used combinations. Combination packaging allows women greater convenience when using either continuous or cyclic estrogen-progesterone regimens. More recently introduced are oral hormonal combinations utilizing the synthetic estrogens and progestins developed for use in birth control pills (ethinyl estradiol plus norethindrone acetate); these combinations are also available for transdermal use. Vaginal rings containing both estrogen and progesterone are currently being investigated for use both in vaginal atrophy and for systemic hormone therapy (Maruo et al. 2002).

Androgens

Data are clear that androgens have mood-enhancing properties and suppress hot flashes in men who have been treated with gonadal suppression. The data in women are much less clear. Estrogen-plus-androgen therapy has been reported to increase libido, decrease breast tenderness, and decrease

TABLE 7–5. Commonly used estrogen+progestin combinations

Brand name (U.S. or Canada)	Estrogen	Progestin	Route
Activella	Estradiol 1 mg	Norethindrone 0.5 mg	1 tablet daily
CombiPatch, Estalis	Estradiol 0.05 mg	Norethindrone 0.25–0.5 mg	Twice-weekly patch
Estratest, Syntest DS	Esterified estrogen 1.25 mg	Methyltestosterone 2.5 mg	1 tablet daily
Estratest HS, Syntest HS	Esterified estrogen 0.625 mg	Methyltestosterone 1.25 mg	1 tablet daily
FemHRT	Ethinyl estradiol 5 µg	Norethindrone 1 mg	1 tablet daily
Prefest	Estradiol 1 mg (every day)	Norgestimate 0.9 mg (3 days on/3 days off)	1 tablet daily
Premphase	Conjugated estrogen 0.626 mg (every day)	Medroxyprogesterone 5 mg (14 days)	1 tablet daily
Prempro, PremPlus	Conjugated estrogen, various doses (every day)	Medroxyprogesterone, various doses (every day)	1 tablet daily

Note. Combination vaginal rings are in clinical trials and will soon be available. Oral contraceptives are used as combination treatment for some perimenopausal women.

the frequency of migraine headaches. A subpopulation of women appears intolerant of androgen therapy, developing marked irritability and depressed mood. Some adverse symptoms are probably dose related, with a greater incidence of side effects seen at higher doses. Side effects secondary to androgen use in women include acne, hirsutism, voice changes, and weight gain; it may also produce an undesirable change in lipid profiles, theoretically enhancing the risk of coronary artery disease (Castelo-Branco et al. 2000).

Combination estrogen plus methyltestosterone is available in two different doses. In clinical practice, the lower dose appears to produce fewer side effects and less discontinuation of treatment. Topical androgen preparations are commonly used for men, and research about appropriate dosing for women with androgen deficiency is under way. Until good data are available, monthly liver function tests and periodic assays for free testosterone should be considered for women using these products off-label.

Antidepressants

Newer antidepressants that affect the release and uptake of serotonin and norepinephrine have become the most promising class of medications for nonhormonal treatment of hot flashes. Venlafaxine, fluoxetine, and paroxetine have been found to reduce hot flashes significantly (by 50%–60%) when compared to placebo. An amino acid analogue, gabapentin, is also showing promise, and randomized controlled trials of its effectiveness are under way. Trials of clonidine have demonstrated a modest, statistically significant reduction in hot flashes, but the benefit was tempered by adverse effects (dry mouth, constipation, drowsiness, and insomnia; Shanafelt et al. 2002).

Selective Estrogen Receptor Modulators

Selective estrogen receptor modulators (SERMs) are a class of synthetic estrogen look-alikes that can act as agonists or antagonists in different tissues. See Table 7–6 for SERMs currently available in the United States. The ideal SERM would provide osteoporosis protection, enhance lipid function, and treat menopausal symptoms (including mood and memory) without increasing risks of breast or endometrial cancer. Unfortunately, currently available drugs in this class appear to provide lipid and bony protection but do not relieve hot flashes (and may transiently make flashes worse).

Tamoxifen is the oldest SERM. Initially used as adjuvant therapy for node-negative breast cancer and therapy for metastatic breast cancer, it is now FDA approved for "reduction in breast cancer incidence in high-risk women." Anecdotal reports of mood deterioration after starting tamoxifen have been reported, but randomized controlled trials are lacking. Raloxifene

TABLE 7–6. Selective estrogen receptor modulators

Generic name	Brand names (U.S. or Canada)	Usual dose	Route
Raloxifene	Evista	60 mg daily	Oral
Tamoxifen[a]	Nolvadex, Tamone	20 mg daily	Oral

Note. Progestin is not required with these agents, even in women with an intact uterus.

[a]Not used for hormone therapy. Used for breast cancer prevention.

was introduced in the United States and Canada for osteoporosis prevention in 1998. It appears to be mood neutral, with the first published study noting "no significant differences between raloxifene groups and the placebo group at any assessment point" (Nickelson et al. 1999). Several other SERMs are currently under development or in clinical trials. See Chapter 3, Effects of Reproductive Hormones and Selective Estrogen Receptor Modulators on the Central Nervous System During Menopause, and Chapter 6, Medical Aspects of Perimenopause and Menopause, for further information on SERMs.

Complementary and Alternative Therapies

See Table 7–7 for complementary and alternative therapies for perimenopausal symptoms. Phytoestrogens are weak estrogens of plant origin that are widely used by perimenopausal women. These compounds are found in soy protein, garbanzo beans, and other legumes (Taylor 2003). Epidemiologic data indicate that women in cultures with high dietary phytoestrogen consumption have fewer menopausal complaints. However, a woman would need to consume a very high daily volume of soy protein, equivalent to six to eight servings of silken tofu, to achieve even slight symptomatic relief (Taylor 2003). There are anecdotal reports of decreased vasomotor symptoms in women using soy products, including dietary supplements, but the results from larger trials are inconsistent or negative (Tice et al. 2003). Beneficial effects on bone mass and cardiovascular disease have been demonstrated in small trials; the role of phytoestrogens in endometrial cancer and mood improvement is unknown (Lichtman 1996).

Ginseng is widely used by perimenopausal women for improving energy and relieving hot flashes. It contains an active ingredient that is chemically similar to estrogen. Mood side effects including nervousness and insomnia have been reported. Hypertension, diarrhea, and vaginal bleeding have also been reported (Seidl and Stewart 1998).

Dang Qui (multiple spellings in the literature) is the most common Chinese herbal for "female complaints," but in clinical testing it has shown no

TABLE 7-7. Complementary therapies for perimenopausal symptoms

Supplement	Symptom	Typical dose	Efficacy and level of evidence[a]
Black cohosh	Hot flash, night sweats	40 mg bid	Possible, C
Chasteberry	Mood changes	30–40 mg daily	Unlikely, C
Calcium	[Osteoporosis prevention]	1,500 mg daily	Yes, B
Dang Qui	"Female complaints"	Variable	Unlikely, C
Evening primrose oil	Hot flashes	2–3 g daily	Unlikely, C
Exercise	[Osteoporosis prevention]	—	Yes, B
Ginkgo biloba	Memory, concentration	80 mg bid	Possible, B
Ginseng root	Hot flashes, low energy	1–2 g daily	Possible, C
Massage	Mood changes	—	Yes, B
Phytoestrogens (soy)	Hot flashes	1–3 g daily	Mixed results, B
	[Osteoporosis prevention]	1–3 g daily	Unlikely, C
Relaxation response	Hot flashes, anxiety	—	Possible, C
St. John's wort	Mood changes	300 mg tid	Possible, B
Valerian root	Sleep disturbances	2–3 g daily	Yes, C

[a]Evidence level A: Large high-quality, randomized, double-blind, placebo-controlled trials, meta-analysis.
Evidence level B: Lesser-quality randomized trials, retrospective studies, systematic reviews.
Evidence level C: Expert opinion, case series, uncontrolled studies, consensus statements.

estrogenic changes in the endometrium or vagina. In double-blind trials, it was no better than placebo for perimenopausal symptoms (Lichtman 1996). It contains numerous coumarin derivatives and is contraindicated in women with increased menstrual bleeding and women using aspirin or anticoagulants (Seidl and Stewart 1998).

Cimicifuga racemosa (black cohosh, squawroot) was widely used by Native American women and was a primary constituent of Lydia Pinkham's Compound. Black cohosh binds estrogen receptors and suppresses LH but not FSH (Lichtman 1996). Clinically, it appears to have some estrogen-like activity, and several clinical trials are in progress. Overall, it has not been shown to reduce hot flashes in a randomized controlled trial in women with a history of breast cancer (Jacobson et al. 2001). Its effect on mood is unknown.

Chasteberry, so named in bygone years because it was used in monasteries to maintain chastity among the monks, stimulates two of the dopamine receptors, has antiandrogenic effects, and inhibits prolactin secretion in vitro. One study has shown effectiveness for treatment of premenstrual symptoms, but data about use in menopause are lacking. Side effects include itching, gastrointestinal symptoms, and headaches (Blumenthal 1998; Seidl and Stewart 1998).

Valeriana officinalis (valerian root) does not have estrogenic properties but has been used for hundreds of years as a sedative and sleep aid in perimenopausal women. The active ingredient is probably a γ-aminobutyric acid (GABA)–like compound. It appears to have limited toxicity and degrades rapidly (Blumenthal 1998). In Germany, valerian root is often used in combination with black cohosh by perimenopausal women.

Vitamin E has shown limited ability to reduce hot flashes, but its documented role as an antioxidant makes it a common choice for perimenopausal women. Vitamin E is contraindicated in women using digitalis or anticoagulants.

Vitamin B_6 has been recommended to improve mood in women with premenstrual dysphoria, but data are mixed, with double-blind trials showing performance equal to placebo. A potential role for improvement of mood in perimenopausal women has been suggested but remains unverified.

Exercise improves both mood and bone mass in perimenopausal women. Relaxation modalities may improve a sense of well-being, but they have no consistently verifiable effects on hot flashes.

Conclusion

The complexities of midlife changes and the management of symptoms related to the menopausal transition make it imperative that gynecologists and mental health professionals work together to meet women's health needs. New research is needed in both medical and psychiatric areas to clarify strategies for the use of hormones in the perimenopause, in contrast to post-menopause studies like the WHI.

References

Avis NE, Stellato R, Crawford S, et al: Is there an association between menopause status and sexual functioning? Menopause 7:297–309, 2000

Birge SJ: Brain aging and estrogens: implications for the care of the postmenopausal woman. Menopause Management July/August:13–21, 2000

Blumenthal M (ed): The Complete German Commission E Monographs. Austin, TX, American Botanical Council, 1998

Brincat M, Kabalan S, Studd JWW, et al: A study of the decrease of skin collagen content, skin thickness, and bone mass in the postmenopausal woman. Obstet Gynecol 70:840–845, 1987

Byyny RL, Speroff L: A Clinical Guide for the Care of Older Women, 2nd Edition. Baltimore, MD, Williams & Wilkins, 1996, pp 143–160

Castelo-Branco C, Vicente JJ, Figueras F, et al: Comparative effects of estrogens plus androgens and tibolone on bone, lipid pattern and sexuality in postmenopausal women. Maturitas 34:161–168, 2000

Dennerstein L, Dudley E, Burger H: Are changes in sexual functioning during midlife due to aging or menopause? Fertil Steril 76:456–460, 2001

Derman RJ, Dawood MY, Stone S: Quality of life during sequential hormone replacement therapy—a placebo-controlled study. Int J Fertil Menopausal Stud 40:73–78, 1995

Erlik Y, Tataryn IV, Meldrum DR, et al: Association of waking episodes with menopausal hot flushes. JAMA 245:1741–1744, 1981

Ginsburg ES: Hot flashes: physiology, hormonal therapy, and alternative therapies. Obstet Gynecol Clin North Am 21:381–390, 1994

Gold EB, Sternfeld B, Kelsey JL, et al: Relation of demographic and lifestyle factors to symptoms in a multi-racial/ethnic population of women 40–55 years of age. Am J Epidemiol 152:463–473, 2000

Gold EB, Block G, Crawford S, et al: Lifestyle and demographic factors in relation to vasomotor symptoms: baseline results from the Study of Women's Health Across the Nation. Am J Epidemiol 159:1189–1199, 2004

Grimes DA, Lobo RA: Perspectives on the Women's Health Initiative trial of hormone replacement therapy. Obstet Gynecol 100:1344–1353, 2002

Grodstein F, Fretts R, Lifford K, et al: Association of age, race, and obstetric history with urinary symptoms among women in the Nurses' Health Study. Am J Obstet Gynecol 189:428–434, 2003

Jacobson JS, Troxel AB, Evans J, et al: Randomized trials of black cohosh for the treatment of hot flashes among women with a history of breast cancer. J Clin Oncol 19:2739–2745, 2001

Kronenberg F: Hot flashes: epidemiology and physiology. Ann N Y Acad Sci 592:52–86, 1990

Lichtman R: Perimenopausal and postmenopausal hormone replacement therapy, part 2: hormonal regimens and complementary and alternative therapies. J Nurse Midwifery 41:195–210, 1996

Lock M: Menopause: lessons from anthropology. Psychosom Med 60:410–419, 1998

Loprinzi CL, Barton DL, Rhodes D: Management of hot flashes in breast cancer survivors. Lancet Oncol 2:199–204, 2001

Maruo T, Mishell DR, Ben-Chetrit A, et al: Vaginal rings delivering progesterone and estradiol may be a new method of hormone replacement therapy. Fertil Steril 78:1010–1016, 2002

Newton KM, LaCroix AZ, Leveille SG, et al: Women's beliefs and decisions about hormone replacement therapy. J Womens Health 6:459–465, 1997

Newton KM, Buist DSM, Keenan NL, et al: Use of alternative therapies for menopause symptoms: results of a population-based survey. Obstet Gynecol 100:18–25, 2002

Nickelson T, Lufkin EG, Riggs BL, et al: Raloxifene hydrochloride, a selective estrogen receptor modulator: safety assessment of effects on cognitive function and mood in postmenopausal women. Psychoneuroendocrinology 24:115–128, 1999

Polo-Kantola P, Erkkola R, Helenius H, et al: When does estrogen replacement therapy improve sleep quality? Am J Obstet Gynecol 178:1002–1009, 1998

Robinson G: Cross-cultural perspectives on menopause. J Nerv Ment Dis 184:453–458, 1996

Sarrel PM: Effects of hormone replacement therapy on sexual psychophysiology and behavior in postmenopause. J Womens Health Gend Based Med 9 (suppl 1):S25–S32, 2000

Scharf MB, McDannold MD, Stover R, et al: Effects of estrogen replacement therapy on rates of cyclic alternating patterns and hot-flush events during sleep in postmenopausal women: a pilot study. Clin Ther 19:304–311, 1997

Schiff I, Regestein Q, Schinfeld J, et al: Interactions of oestrogens and hours of sleep on cortisol, FSH, LH, and prolactin in hypogonadal women. Maturitas 2:179–183, 1980

Seidl MM, Stewart DE: Alternative treatments for menopausal symptoms. Can Fam Physician 44:1299–1308, 1998

Shanafelt T, Barton D, Adjei A, et al: Pathophysiology and treatment of hot flashes. Mayo Clin Proc 77:1207–1218, 2002

Shaywitz SE, Shaywitz BA, Pugh KR, et al: Effect of estrogen on brain activation patterns in postmenopausal women during working memory tasks. JAMA 281:1197–1202, 1999

Sherwin BB: The impact of different doses of estrogen and progestin on mood and sexual behavior in postmenopausal women. J Clin Endocrinol Metab 72:336–343, 1991

Sherwin BB: Menopause myths and realities, in Psychological Aspects of Women's Health Care: The Interface Between Psychiatry and Obstetrics and Gynecology, 2nd Edition. Edited by Stotland NL, Stewart DE. Washington, DC, American Psychiatric Press, 2001, pp 241–259

Sherwin BB, Tulandi T: "Add-back" estrogen reverses cognitive deficits induced by a gonadotropin-releasing hormone agonist in women with leiomyomata uteri. J Clin Endocrinol Metab 81:2545–2549, 1996

Speroff L, Glass RH, Kase NG: Clinical Gynecologic Endocrinology and Infertility, 6th Edition. Baltimore, MD, Lippincott Williams & Wilkins, 1999, pp 643–724

Stanton AL, Lobel M, Sears S, et al: Psychosocial aspects of selected issues in women's reproductive health: current status and future directions. J Consult Clin Psychol 70:751–770, 2002

Stearns V, Beebe KL, Iyengar M, et al: Paroxetine controlled release in the treatment of menopausal hot flashes. JAMA 289:2827–2834, 2003

Taylor M: Alternatives to HRT: an evidence-based review. Int J Fertil Womens Med 48:64–68, 2003

Tice JA, Ettinger B, Ensrud K, et al: Phytoestrogen supplements for the treatment of hot flashes: the Isoflavone Clover Extract (ICE) Study: a randomized controlled trial. JAMA 290:207–214, 2003

Utian WH: Semantics, menopause-related terminology, and the STRAW reproductive aging staging system. Menopause 8:398–401, 2001

Versi E, Harvey M-A, Cardozo L, et al: Urogenital prolapse and atrophy at menopause: a prevalence study. Int Urogynecol J Pelvic Floor Dysfunct 12:107–110, 2001

Willhite LA, O'Connell MD: Urogenital atrophy: prevention and treatment. Pharmacotherapy 21:464–480, 2001

Women's Health Initiative Study Group: Design of the Women's Health Initiative clinical trial and observational study. Control Clin Trials 19:61–109, 1998

Writing Group for the PEPI Trial: Effects of estrogen or estrogen/progestin regimens on heart disease risk factors in postmenopausal women. The Postmenopausal Estrogen/Progestin Interventions (PEPI) Trial. JAMA 273:199–208, 1995

Writing Group for the Women's Health Initiative Investigators: Risks and benefits of estrogen plus progestin in healthy postmenopausal women: principal results from the Women's Health Initiative randomized controlled trial. JAMA 288:321–333, 2002

Chapter 8

Beyond Menopause

The Psychopathology and Psychotherapy of Older Women

Marta B. Rondon, M.D.

*O*n average, women live longer than men. Once the changes of perimenopause are over, a woman can expect her life to extend for a significant period, with life spans increasing almost everywhere in the world. It is not easy to define *older*. The term generally refers to people older than 60 years. Unfortunately, it often carries negative connotations, conjuring up images of disability and dementia, implying that older people are dependent and need to be "looked after." This popular notion means that policy planners and caregivers tend to disregard the opinions and wishes of older people—especially those of elderly women who are disempowered as a result of not only advanced age but also their female gender and, often, low income.

Even given an agreed-upon definition of *older,* one must remember that not all women over age 60 are equal. The disparities and experiences of earlier years may be amplified throughout life. Furthermore, once a woman is deemed to be old, it is often hard to make sure that she will not have to face further discrimination and inequitable treatment.

Cultural Factors

In developing countries, older women are often responsible for transmitting cultural mores and values to younger members of the community. They also take care of youngsters orphaned by war, AIDS, or other catastrophes, and they hold families together in troubled times. But when resources are scarce, women past their reproductive years are certainly not a priority. Older women are especially vulnerable in situations of poverty and inequality and during disasters.

There is less discrimination against older people in developed regions, at least with regard to accessing services. However, the materialistic lifestyle of many developed societies and the breakdown of spiritual networks have eroded family cohesiveness, so that older women frequently face loneliness, isolation, and the prospect of spending their final years in nursing homes.

Even in regions such as Nepal, where religious traditions still include reverence for the elderly, social and economic pressures are forcing the young to move away from their villages, leaving their elders at the mercy of neighbors and relatives who may consider them burdensome, inactive, and useless recipients of valuable support (Swar 2003). Because of the economic hardship, older people are subject to abandonment and discrimination even in the most traditional settings.

The healthy aging of women poses a major challenge for both developed and developing nations. Although about 135 million women over age 60 inhabit developed areas, more than 198 million live in developing regions, and two-thirds of the world's women ages 45–59 years also live in developing countries (World Health Organization 2002a).

Longer lives are not necessarily healthier lives. In all regions of the world, more women than men can expect to spend some part of their lives with certain limitations. This is not to say that all older women are frail, nor that they must invariably expect to be sick in their old age. But it certainly challenges the medical profession to identify the determinants of healthy aging and to find ways to ensure that those who suffer from diseases and limitations receive appropriate, good-quality health care.

Determinants of Health in Older Women

Factors known to influence the health of women as they age include poverty, education, gender-based division of domestic chores, violence, abuse, and access to health insurance and paid employment in formal sectors.

Poverty and unhealthy aging are inextricably intertwined, especially when years of childbearing and dietary deprivation leave older women with nutritional deficits and weak bones. Cognitive losses may be amplified by the physical and mental consequences of long-term exposure to household toxins, agricultural pesticides, and polluted water.

The type and extent of education play a dominant role in determining health disparities between populations. Education is closely linked to income, lifestyle, work, job conditions, housing, and opportunities for advancement.

Because domestic chores are usually allocated according to gender, with females bearing the brunt, being responsible for child care and looking after ill relatives, many women must work until they die. Moreover, the increasing participation of young women in the labor force, along with shorter hospitalization stays as a result of managed care and other cost-cutting policies, pushes an ever-growing share of child care onto older women. These tasks can seriously undermine physical and psychological well-being.

Women as Caregivers

Caring for sick relatives frequently puts a woman at risk for depressive and anxiety symptoms, robbing her of autonomy and the ability to look after herself. Anticipatory grief may also need to be faced, just when there are already severe demands on the woman's time and energy. The fact that caring for relatives is perceived as part of a woman's natural gender-based duties makes it still more burdensome. This is well illustrated by the contrast between women caring for sick relatives, who often consider the task onerous and harmful to psychological and physical health, and voluntary or paid caregivers, who often find the job rewarding (Paoletti 1999).

Theorists propose that greater centrality (personal control) in social roles enhances psychological well-being, but also that role centrality exacerbates the negative effects of stress. Support for both hypotheses comes from studies of 296 women who simultaneously adopted the roles of mother, wife, parent care provider, and employee. Greater control in all four roles improved psychological well-being. But, as predicted, depressive symptoms arose when too much emphasis was put on controlling aspects of domestic life, as was the case with women who were wives, mothers, and workers at the same time. Contrary to expectations, focusing on the mother role seemed to buffer the negative stress of multiple roles. These findings suggest that performing multiple roles may be protective against depression (Martire et al. 2000).

Studies show that 80% of U.S. caregivers are the spouses of homeowners, and most are women. Women may find themselves caring for their spouses, in-laws, and children. They might spend up to 13 hours a day providing care and might continue to do so for more than 20 years (Bradley 2003). Roughly half of these female caregivers report poor or fair health, and one-third say that their health has deteriorated in the past 6 months. About 80% have unmet health needs, and 25% require education about diseases that afflict their relatives.

Providing care for a frail older adult is frequently viewed as a stressful experience that erodes psychological well-being and physical health. In a recent meta-analysis (Pinquart and Sorensen 2003), the authors integrated findings from 84 articles on differences between caregivers and noncaregivers in terms of perceived stress, depression, general subjective well-being, physical health, and self-efficacy. Caregivers were found to have more depression and stress and less of a sense of self-efficacy, as well as lower general subjective well-being. Differences in the levels of physical health in favor of noncaregivers were statistically significant but small. However, larger differences were found between caregivers and noncaregivers of dementia patients than were found between heterogeneous samples of caregivers and noncaregivers.

Data from the Nurses' Health Study indicate that women who provided 36 or more weekly hours of care to a disabled spouse were almost six times more likely than noncaregivers to experience depressive or anxiety symptoms. Looking after a disabled or ill parent produced less dramatic elevations in depressive or anxiety symptoms (Cannuscio et al. 2002).

It is already well established that caregiver stress affects women regardless of age or ethnicity (Wallace Williams et al. 2003). In a group of Korean women, the relationship to the patient did not alter the negative impact of caregiving (Kim 2001).

Bergs (2002) examined the emotional status of women caring for patients with chronic obstructive pulmonary disease. The women ranged in age from 47 to 69 years. Wives who had given up work because of spousal illness complained about curtailed recreation and lack of support from friends, families, and health care providers. Sherif et al. (2001) reported that caregivers of nondepressed oncology patients showed above-average levels of depressive symptoms on the Hamilton Rating Scale for Depression.

Caring for relatives with mental illness seems to be particularly difficult. One study found that 25% of women caring for schizophrenic patients had General Health Questionnaire scores indicating stress burdens compatible with psychiatric cases (Laidlaw et al. 2002). Similarly, depression was more common among caregivers of spouses with Alzheimer's disease (AD) than among those caring for people with Parkinson's disease (without dementia) (Hooker et al. 1998). However, some caregivers also report positive aspects of caring for mentally ill family members (Veltman et al. 2002).

Women, Work, and Health Care

Because many women work in informal sectors, as part-timers or in family businesses, they are more likely than men to lack proper pension plans and health insurance, hampering their ability to receive appropriate health care. For women over age 60, the consequences of inadequate care may mean neglect in treating common emotional disorders, failure to detect early-stage malignancies and heart disease, poor management, and premature death. Close to 60% of all adult female deaths are because of heart disease or stroke (World Health Organization 2002b).

Even if an older woman does receive health care, the care often leaves much to be desired and may be of inferior quality. Older women, in particular, are overprescribed sedatives and hypnotics that may lead to habituation, cognitive dulling, and increased tendency to falls. Improper diagnosis, failure to pinpoint the origins and cause of a problem, and disregard for the slower metabolic processes and use of concurrent drugs in older patients can easily lead to inappropriate prescription, adverse drug reactions, and multiple drug interactions.

A Swedish study of women ages 55–65 years found more morbidity in postmenopausal than in premenopausal women. The most prevalent complaints were musculoskeletal joint problems and headaches. Vaginal dryness and hot flashes were clearly linked to menopause, and 85% of the sample also reported psychological symptoms (Li et al. 2002).

The complaints of a group of 204 women with coronary artery disease about the poor care received and limitations encountered during rehabilitation illustrate common obstacles facing older women. Most of the study participants were on multiple medications and had unsatisfactory relationships with their health care providers, chiefly because of communication problems bad enough to inhibit them from asking about their disease and its treatment options. Many women said they were unable or unwilling to make appropriate lifestyle changes after diagnosis because of insufficient social, medical, or educational support. Less than 60% were offered rehabilitation services. Most reported financial hardships because of their disease. This sample highlights the failure to fulfill the needs of older women for good-quality, readily available health services that can maintain functional competence (Marcuccio et al. 2003).

Postmenopausal Women and Exercise

Functional competence is the degree to which individuals manage to think, feel, and behave in harmony with their environment and energy reserves.

Functional competence involves emotional health, self-esteem, intellectual status, social activity, and attitudes toward oneself and the world. It determines the extent to which a woman can cope independently and within the community. Functional ability may decrease after menopause because of fatigue, anemia, osteoporosis, joint pain, thyroid disorders, obesity, heart disease, stroke, and other conditions. Impaired or restricted mobility is the most frequent ailment found in women over age 60, both in developed and developing nations.

It is common knowledge that passive, sedentary lifestyles lead to poor physical health and reduced functional capacity. Research confirms that physical activity protects people against many diseases, including cardiovascular ailments and conditions affecting mobility. It also improves their balance and diminishes the risk of falls and consequent fractures. Staying active and continuing to exercise are the most significant means by which people can improve their health status (World Health Organization 1998).

Aging inevitably brings some concerns about the aging person's independence, health, and functional competence. By helping to maintain functional competence and independence, physical activity can also protect emotional well-being and strengthen coping skills. In all parts of the world, exercise and physical activity exert a beneficial impact throughout the life span. It is therefore essential that every effort be made to educate women of all ages and help them understand the health benefits of physical and recreational activities. Any cultural or social barriers that hamper or prevent girls from exercising should be avoided or abolished. In addition, women should be encouraged to maintain an appropriate body weight by adopting healthy eating habits and should be discouraged from smoking by all available means.

Empowerment of younger women is a key element in building healthy self-esteem throughout life. Such empowerment must be strongly fostered so that women become better equipped to handle events and crises in later years, such as widowhood, chronic illness, and the ensuing disabilities and financial hardships.

Violence Against the Older Woman

Although its impact is often ignored or neglected, violence is a dominant threat for the older woman. Because of their frequently inferior social standing, as well as economic and political disadvantages, older women frequently suffer abuse and discrimination at the hands of relatives, communities, states, and agencies charged with their protection. Women with cognitive impairment are especially vulnerable to violence and to economic and emotional abuse. The effects of violence against women in several parts of the world have been amply illustrated through consultations held by HelpAge International ("Gender and Aging Briefs" 2000). These consultations revealed that women in Eastern Europe were mainly worried about street crime; those in Latin America complained of intergenerational conflict, forced displacement, disrespectful treatment, and social violence; and older women in the Caribbean were distressed about beatings received at the hands of relatives who were under the influence of drugs or were collecting money for drug consumption. In Africa, witchcraft accusations were cited as a serious form of violence against women, resulting in the deaths of several hundred victims every year. In many parts of the world, traditional dresses that completely cover a woman's body hamper her freedom of movement, making her more vulnerable to assault, particularly if she also suffers from one or more of the mobility limitations common in older women. Such garments may also hide wounds received through violence in the home.

Sexual abuse seems to be widespread in regions where women are left without partners, be it through war or abandonment. The perpetrator is usually a member of the household, although women with cognitive deficits may be abused by caregivers. Acts of violence and abuse against older women often remain unreported because of shame and denial, ignorance of the victim's rights, and fear of reprisal.

Violence against the older woman is the ultimate expression and consequence of the lack of power and representation. The characteristics that make women especially liable to abuse are strongly gender related, depicting the huge power gap between males and females and between generations.

Psychopathology Beyond Menopause

Depression and dementia are among the top 10 causes of morbidity and mortality among women in the Americas (Bonita 2003). Because these conditions are somewhat similar but have different origins and outcomes, differential diagnosis is essential. However, the passivity that accompanies depression in older women often hinders its recognition.

Depression

As at other life stages in most regions, depression continues to be more prevalent with advancing years among women than men. There are various reasons for this discrepancy. According to a biopsychosocial susceptibility model, women are more prone to depression because of genetic predisposition, greater exposure to stressful life events, and modulation of the neuroendocrine system in response to fluctuating gonadal hormone levels.

There is increasing evidence that the neuroendocrine molecule estradiol-17β plays a role in younger women's depressive states. In the older woman, an accumulation of lifetime stressors, together with the decline in ovarian function, nutritional deficits, and lifestyle factors, may interact with physical limitations and a past history of depression to create and maintain high rates of this illness.

Milder forms of depression often go unrecognized and untreated. For management of depression in elderly patients, female gender predicates a bad prognosis, especially if the depression is accompanied by negative experiences, living alone, poor physical condition, and few social contacts (Denihan et al. 2000).

Depression may cause or exacerbate physical illness in older women. Chronic depression predisposes one to osteoporosis and worsens the prognosis of ischemic heart disease (Frasure-Smith et al. 1995). At the same time, ill health plays a crucial role in the genesis and persistence of depression. Many women over age 60 suffer from mobility impairment, heart disease, stroke, cancer (lung, breast, and cervical), diabetes, nutritional deficits, anemia, obesity, poor balance, sensory impairment (hearing and visual losses), and other conditions. However, some somatic symptoms described by postmenopausal women may stem from the depression. See Chapter 6, Medical Aspects of Perimenopause and Menopause, for physical illnesses that may be associated with menopause.

Bereavement in widows is strongly related to their high rates of depression and ill health. In fact, loss of a partner is rated as the single most significant life event that triggers persistent depression. Widowhood usually entails a change in status and living arrangements. Lack of control over choice, rather than the choice itself, seems most likely to induce depressive symptoms.

The relevance of social support to the prognosis of depression remains controversial. Some authors report that unsatisfactory and infrequent contacts are related to depression (Henderson et al. 1997), whereas others find no such link.

It is well established that severe depression in the elderly increases mortality risks. However, it seems that milder forms of depression do not necessarily raise mortality risks in women but rather increase morbidity. Using the patients in the Amsterdam Study of the Elderly, Schoevers et al. (2000) found that although 75% of men suffering from psychotic depression were dead at follow-up (6 years after diagnosis), 53.6% of women with psychotic depression were alive after 6 years. In men, the presence of neurotic depression doubled mortality from 30.3% (without depression) to 59.3%. However, in women the presence of neurotic depression raised mortality insignificantly, from 20.5% to 23.1%. Prevalence of depression at baseline was 12.9% overall (neurotic, 10.9%; psychotic, 2.0%), 6.9% in men, and 16.5% in women. Because functional disability frequently results from or follows depression, and the number of men with psychotic depression was rather small, it seems reasonable to conclude that psychotic depression produces a higher risk of mortality for both sexes. However, gender differences were most apparent when investigating the more prevalent neurotic depression. Neurotic depression in women was not significantly linked with mortality.

There is also a distinct possibility that depression in later years may be a risk factor or even a prodrome for dementia. Geerlings et al. (2000) examined data from the 4,051 participants in the Amsterdam Study of the Elderly and the 3,107 participants in the Longitudinal Aging Study Amsterdam. They found that depression was associated with elevated risks of AD and cognitive decline only in people with high educational levels. This apparent link between depression and educational achievement requires further study to fully understand this finding, as intellectually active people are usually less at risk for dementia. Neurochemical and neuropathological studies on the brains of AD patients suggest that these people may have a decreased threshold for depression and that the dementia process itself may contribute to depression. In fact, depression as an early symptom of dementia might be more obviously recognizable in highly educated individuals. Furthermore, the more severely depressed older people were at greater risk of developing cognitive losses in the Longitudinal Aging Study Amsterdam group, suggesting a possible biological relationship between depression and dementia.

One potential mechanism is that depression is associated with high levels of cortisol, which may cause neuronal death, especially in the hippocampus and hypothalamus (Herbert 1998).

Anxiety

Although not mentioned among the more severe mental health problems of older women, anxiety disorders are the cause of significant suffering and reduction in the quality of life in this population, even more so than asthma or cardiac disease. Generalized anxiety disorder commonly accompanies depression in women during later life (Xavier et al. 2003).

Anxiety is often related to ill health and the accompanying pain, loss of function, and impending death. Sometimes anxiety is not diagnosed, and the symptoms (palpitations, dyspnea, dizziness) are attributed to an exacerbation of an underlying medical illness (such as thyroid disease), a change in living circumstances (such as a hospital admission), or surgery. Conversely, several conditions and many medications may cause secondary anxiety. The symptoms of anxiety can also result from a medical illness, complicating the differential diagnosis.

Older people often receive prescriptions for hypnotics and sedatives. A woman is 2.5 times as likely to receive an anxiolytic as a man, and 3% of all women over age 60 receive medication for anxiety, resulting in a risk of dependency on benzodiazepines (Stein and Barrett-Connor 2002).

Personal anxiety toward aging is related to anxiety about death and societal attitudes toward aging. Women seem to be more anxious about death. Higher levels of fear and anxiety about aging, dying, and the unknown, in turn, are found in people who regard older age as less valued socially (DePaola et al. 2003).

Phobic anxiety is fairly common among elderly people. Agoraphobia is common in elderly women and can be exacerbated by admission to a hospital or other traumatic events.

Posttraumatic stress disorder is a chronic condition that can persist into old age, as is exemplified by Holocaust survivors. In older patients, there seem to be fewer reexperiencing symptoms and more hyperactivation symptoms (Deimling et al. 2002).

Both cognitive-behavioral psychotherapy and other approaches have been found useful in the management of anxiety disorders in older women. Further research is needed to provide more alternatives to benzodiazepines and hypnotics in this population in order to avoid habituation and falls leading to fractures.

Obsessive-Compulsive Disorder

The incidence of obsessive-compulsive disorder in older adults is about 0.55 per 1,000 person-years, with a significantly higher incidence in women (Nestadt et al. 1998). In addition to new cases of obsessive-compulsive disorder, some will appear to occur as an exaggeration of a preexisting obsessional personality style.

Obsessive-compulsive disorder is well known in the institutionalized elderly, especially among those with cognitive disturbances. Obsessive religious thoughts and hoarding behaviors are fairly common in older women.

Bipolar Disorder

Bipolar disorder may have its onset after age 60, or it may persist throughout life into older age. Late-onset bipolar disorder has been described as more frequent in women (Almeida and Fenner 2002). Bipolar disorder patients use health services even more than do elderly depressed patients (Charney et al. 2003). However, despite the prevalence, morbidity, and mortality of bipolar disorder in late life, there are very few studies in older populations.

Diagnosis of bipolar disorder is a particularly neglected area, with agitated depression sometimes considered a form of bipolar disorder. A controversy exists regarding the organic nature of late-onset bipolar disorder. Older patients with bipolar disorder are at increased risk for cerebrovascular illness and psychotic features. The assessment of bipolar disorder should include the ruling out of comorbid conditions and medications that may cause mania (e.g., corticosteroids for the management of connective tissue disorders).

Rapid cycling (defined as more than four affective episodes in 1 year) is more common in women than men, frequently begins in perimenopause, and may be linked to the use of antidepressants or hypothyroidism. Rapid cycling persists for several years in 40% of cases, and in 13% it reverts to long cycles.

The pharmacotherapy of bipolar disorder in the older woman has followed the same guidelines as in younger adults, but changes in brain and metabolic function with variations in the pharmacodynamics and pharmacokinetics of psychotropic drugs make this a potentially dangerous strategy.

Mood stabilizers seem to be effective in older people, although there are as yet no controlled studies. Lithium should be administered with caution in older patients because kidney function may be impaired. Moreover, there is a narrow therapeutic dosing range for lithium in the elderly, thus increasing the risk for toxicity. Thyroid function in elderly patients taking lithium should be monitored. Divalproex has received support as an effective and well-tolerated mood stabilizer for geriatric bipolar disorder, particularly in managing acute mania (MacDonald and Nemeroff 1998). There is a lack of controlled trials of psychotherapy, psychoeducation, or other nonpharmacological treatments in the geriatric bipolar population (Shulman et al. 2003).

Personality Disorders

The functioning of older women as well as their response to psychosocial and psychopharmacological treatments is influenced by personality. Axis II disorders have been studied in older depressed populations and in institutionalized people, although there is a lack of community data.

Rigidity and maladaptive functioning persist into older age and get worse as cognitive decline increases. Isolation and the diminished social valuation of older women make narcissistic traits more apparent; the frailty of older age and cognitive difficulties reinforce avoidant and dependent traits as well as low tolerance and irritability. Dependent and avoidant older people seem to have more difficulties with activities of daily living than one would expect.

The presence of personality disorders has been studied in populations of depressed (major and minor) and dysthymic older persons. Personality disorders in late life are associated with poor outcomes, less response to psychotherapies, and suicide. One study of 47 patients who had been treated for major depression looked at the relationship between symptoms of personality disorder and measures of disability, social functioning, and interpersonal relations (Abrams et al. 1998). Schizoid, schizotypal, and paranoid personality pathologies were responsible for slower response to a combination of nortriptyline and interpersonal therapy. Narcissistic, paranoid, and schizoid personality disorders seemed to relate to unsatisfactory interpersonal relationships, and schizoid, schizotypal, avoidant, and narcissistic personality disorders to lower sociability scores. Gender was associated with poor personal relationships and less independent functioning, especially in women with some residual signs of depression.

Devanand et al. (2000) reported that personality disorders, especially obsessive-compulsive and avoidant disorders, affect one-third of late-onset dysthymic patients over 60 years. However, they noted that only 20% of the patients with comorbid Axis II diagnoses are women (Denand et al. 2000).

Borderline personality disorder is linked to suicidality and benzodiazepine abuse in the elderly. In one study, the typical benzodiazepine user was characterized as a widowed woman with dysthymic disorder, anxiety, predisposition to alcohol dependence, and borderline disorder (Petrovic et al. 2002).

A variety of individual and group therapies are useful to promote socialization, acceptance of difficulties, and elaboration of insight in borderline personality disorder patients (Carrasco 2002).

Cognitive Changes, Delirium, and Dementia

Some studies suggest that a longer lifetime exposure to endogenous estrogen may protect against age-related cognitive decline (McLay et al. 2003; Sherwin 1994). However, one must consider the possibility that better-educated, more functionally competent women tend to opt for hormone therapy (Lokkegaard et al. 2002).

In 1996, the Women's Health Initiative Memory Study (WHIMS) began enrolling women participating in the Women's Health Initiative Study, in a large trial of estrogen and progestin in women over 65. The WHIMS was designed to examine the probable protective effect of estrogen on cognitive function, because this issue had been researched before in different settings, with conflicting results. WHIMS results show that among 4,381 women randomized to either 0.625 mg of conjugated equine estrogen plus 2.5 mg of medroxyprogesterone acetate or placebo, more women receiving estrogen had a significantly higher decline in Mini-Mental State Examination scores (6.7%) compared with the placebo group (4.8%). These results do not support the administration of estrogen to women over 65 to protect their cognitive functioning (Rapp et al. 2003).

Delirium

A diagnosis of delirium requires a disturbance of conscience, a change in cognition or perceptual disturbance that develops rapidly and fluctuates during the day and that is related to a medical condition, substance withdrawal or intoxication, or a combination of these (American Psychiatric Association 2000). Delirium is distressing for relatives and patients, is costly to manage, prolongs hospital stay, may not clear immediately after correction of the causing condition, and is significantly related to mortality.

The prevalence of delirium ranges from 11% to 16%, and it is more frequent in people over 60 (Levkoff et al. 1992). Because women live longer than men, they are at increased risk for dementia, hip fracture, urinary tract infections, adverse effects of multiple medications, and undernourishment, leading to a heightened risk of delirium. Elderly patients, and especially women, are extremely sensitive to surgery, anesthesia, drug toxicity, infections, structural brain disease, electrolyte imbalance, and sensory deprivation. In addition, age-related changes in metabolism and pharmacokinetics and pharmacodynamics, deterioration of sight and hearing, and diminished resistance to physical stress make older adults very vulnerable to delirium.

Delirium is a syndrome, not a disease; it represents the common pathway of many potential causes. A careful search for the underlying condition should always be undertaken. The presentation of delirium can mimic functional psychiatric disorders. It may start with a prodromal phase: 2–3 days of malaise, restlessness, poor concentration, anxiety, irritability, sleep disturbances, and nightmares. A consequence of this broad symptom profile is that it may be mistaken for dementia or functional psychiatric disorders. Emotional and behavioral changes of delirium are easily confused with adjustment reactions, particularly in patients who have experienced major trauma or diagnosis of a serious condition. Delirium is frequently confused with depression, especially in women and those with hypoactive or lethargic delirium presentations. Most symptoms of major depression can occur in delirium (e.g., psychomotor slowing, sleep disturbances, and irritability), but the onset of depressive illness is less acute and mood disturbance (rather than disorientation) dominates the clinical picture. Although hypoactive patients are perceived as less morbid, they have poorer outcomes that, in part, reflect poorer identification and less aggressive treatment of delirium. Moreover, the efficacy of antipsychotics in the treatment of patients with both hypoactive and hyperactive profiles is poorly appreciated (Meagher 2001). Mistaking delirium for depression may prompt the clinician to prescribe antidepressants, with the danger of worsening the delirium and delaying appropriate evaluation and management of the underlying primary condition.

The management of delirium involves the diagnosis of the cause or causes of brain disorder that are being expressed as disorientation and confusion. These conditions must be corrected whenever possible and nonpharmacological and pharmacological measures instituted. A restful, quiet room, the company of a familiar person, and consistency of caretaking personnel are useful. Administration of antipsychotic medications, at low doses initially, is the recommended approach.

Dementia: Alzheimer's Disease

Alzheimer's disease is the most common form of dementia, accounting for 50%–70% of all cases. It is a progressive dementia characterized by widespread neuronal loss, β-amyloid deposits, the development of neuritic plaques, and the presence of neurofibrillary tangles. The association areas of the cerebral cortex, the hippocampus, and the middle and temporal lobes are most commonly affected. Also typical of AD is a decrease in acetylcholine levels, paralleling the severity of dementia.

The primary symptoms of AD are declines in memory and cognition, producing a marked and progressive deterioration in daily functioning. Changes in personality may also be noticed as early symptoms of the illness, and behavioral disturbances including agitation, hallucinations, and delusions appear as the disease progresses. The illness lasts approximately 7–10 years from the time of diagnosis until death (Mayeaux 1999).

DSM-IV-TR (American Psychiatric Association 2000) criteria for the clinical diagnosis of probable AD include onset between ages 40 and 90; no disturbance of consciousness; dementia established by clinical examination and a standardized assessment of mental status, supplemented by neuropsychological tests; deficits in two or more areas of cognition (one being memory), characterized by gradual onset and progression; absence of systemic disorders or other brain diseases (such as minor strokes) to explain the progressive decline in memory and cognition; and deficits not exclusively during an episode of delirium.

Risk factors for AD are increasing age, female gender, genetic markers, and a positive family history. The incidence of AD doubles every 5 years over age 60. It is most common in women, although the fact that men are more prone to vascular dementia might preclude them from being counted among those with pure AD (Alzheimer's Association 2003).

As to the genetic risk, less than 5% of AD patients have point mutations in chromosomes 1, 14, and 21. The E4 allele of apolipoprotein E (a protein active in the repair of neurons and in cholesterol transport) is a genetic risk factor for the development of AD. This protein is encoded in chromosome 19, and there are three variants (E2, E3, E4). Subjects who have one E4 allele have a doubled risk of developing AD, and those who are homozygous for the E4 allele have 10 times the risk.

Family history, independent of genetic makeup, is an added risk factor, especially for women. People with first-degree relatives who have the disease have two to four times the average risk of AD. Clearly, genetics and family history interact, so the risk for a woman who has both genetic markers and a first-degree relative with the disease is extremely high.

Other suggested risk factors include traumatic head injury, depression, low levels of educational and occupational attainment, and disinterest or low participation in social activities, although some of these factors may stem from socioeconomic factors.

Because postmenopausal women have a higher risk of developing AD, it has been hypothesized that decreasing estrogen levels might be involved. The neuroprotective effects of estrogen are well known. See Chapter 3, Effects of Reproductive Hormones and Selective Estrogen Receptor Modulators on the Central Nervous System During Menopause. As previously stated, several studies have been carried out, some showing a lower risk of AD for women receiving estrogen replacement, but prospective studies fail to show similar results. Particularly significant in this regard is the WHIMS (mentioned earlier), designed to evaluate the effect of estrogen with or without progestin versus placebo on 1) all causes of dementia, 2) mild cognitive impairment (MCI), and 3) global cognitive functioning. Women without dementia or MCI participating in the WHI were eligible. In total, of the 4,532 women participating, 40 in the estrogen/progestin group and 21 in the placebo group (61 total) were diagnosed with dementia during the trial. Twice as many women in the estrogen/progestin group were diagnosed with dementia, mostly of the Alzheimer type. Of the group receiving estrogen/progestin, 61 were diagnosed with MCI not followed by dementia; 11 with MCI followed by probable dementia; and 29 with probable dementia not preceded by MCI; compared with 45, 10, and 11, respectively, in the placebo group.

These results demonstrate that estrogen with or without progestin does not protect postmenopausal women against MCI, and furthermore, it increases the risk of dementia (Shumaker et al. 2003).

Psychotherapy

Given the high prevalence of mild to moderate depressive disorders in older women and the difficulties of managing them psychopharmacologically, several authors have explored the value of psychotherapy for postmenopausal women. The therapies that seem to be most effective for older adults include cognitive-behavioral treatment of sleep disorders and psychodynamic, cognitive, interpersonal, and behavioral treatments for clinical depression. Memory retraining and cognitive training are sometimes efficacious in slowing cognitive decline in nonsyndromal problems of aging.

Preliminary evidence suggests that psychotherapy not only can reduce psychopathology but may also alleviate physical complaints, pain, and disability, perhaps even improving compliance with medical regimens. Psychotherapy has been found most effective in treating depression related to bereavement and caregiver burden (Klausner and Alexopoulos 1999).

Diverse types of psychotherapy, described next, can prove useful for older women, depending on the therapist's skills and patient characteristics.

The basic *psychodynamic* assumption that symptoms and personality problems have hidden and unconscious meanings, that a developmental process exists, and that each person has a complex inner world applies equally to older and younger individuals. Erikson's model of epigenetic development helps us understand the elderly condition: The developmental task of this age is to negotiate between ego-integrity and ego-despair. Integrity consists of valuing one's own life experience, holding on to the worthwhile aspects of one's life, and retaining memories of having been valued and loved. Ego-despair arises through a sense of "not being" and from feelings of disgust at degeneration or loss of faculties. People who have not developed basic trust in early childhood will have more difficulties in accepting the inevitable changes of aging and may develop panic and depression, as well as a terrifying dread of dependency.

Among the many difficulties to surmount in later life are issues with sexuality or loss of sexual attraction or interest; the threat of role displacement, particularly if the role is perceived as central and essential; changes in marital relationships as children leave, marry, or have babies; a sense of having failed as a parent; distress about bodily changes; awareness of the limits to future achievement; loss of a partner or of intimacy through separation, illness, or death; and the probability of one's own death.

Age can be perceived as a narcissistic wound beyond repair, particularly in individuals who equate success with external values or those who over-adapt to socioenvironmental pressures. For such people, dealing with retirement, bereavement, or body changes engenders a sense of futility, alienation, and despair that can easily become overwhelming.

Conversely, the therapeutic relationship might help the woman view age as an opportunity for growth—provided she can call on coping skills and attributes that have previously worked for her. A patient may be helped to appreciate the age-related ability to delay gratification and greater resilience (the capacity to preserve healthy functioning despite adverse life circumstances).

Emotional isolation can be reduced within an intimate and containing therapeutic relationship, provided the psychotherapist pays close attention and takes care to display appropriate psychotherapeutic responses—the ability to listen and empathize, to make sense of the patient's experiences, to contain anxiety and despair rather than feeling compelled to act (prescribe), and to bear hostility and criticism without retaliation—as well as identifying a patient's distorted perception of the relationship (Garner 2002).

Interpersonal therapy (IPT) may also be useful for older women, because menopause and postmenopause involve role transitions, many losses, and isolation. The areas addressed by IPT that are most relevant to older women are high risks of grief and delayed mourning of lost partners and loved ones; role transitions resulting from changes in health, wealth, and employment; altered family roles and dynamics; interpersonal conflicts linked to dependency on others or decisions about where to live; and interpersonal deficits related to long-standing patterns of isolation and loneliness or stemming from decreased energy and motivation.

Adapting IPT to older persons may require greater flexibility, helping both the talkative woman who has difficulty in focusing and the frail patient unable to tolerate a full session. Dependency issues must be analyzed for validity, and the patient should be encouraged to strive for greater independence or to accept the need for help as appropriate. In addressing role disputes, a realistic aim might be to increase the patient's tolerance of the more distressing aspects of a relationship and to facilitate appreciation of any positive aspects. Transference should not be interpreted, just as it is not interpreted in younger patients in IPT, and a neutral stance should be avoided. Specific therapeutic suggestions about ways to increase social contacts are entirely appropriate. The measuring of treatment gains may need to be tailored; some older women may need constant reassurance that they are making progress, whereas others might be satisfied with small gains.

With older women it may be helpful to focus on grief, even though the anticipated death has not yet occurred. Women caring for a severely demented or terminally ill spouse are in fact already grieving the loss of the originally loved person.

In relation to grief, some patients may hide their feelings as they are overwhelmed with responsibility and have no time for themselves, others might have survived severe stress (such as a risky operation of the spouse) only to find themselves overburdened by a minor problem (such as arrangements for a maid), and still others may be trying too hard to avoid depression, thus not allowing themselves to face their own feelings. These circumstances might impede progress in therapy (Frank et al. 1993).

Interpersonal therapy can also be useful as maintenance therapy and may be combined with antidepressant medication (Miller et al. 2001). Maintenance IPT seems to be most effective in women who focus on role conflict rather than in those with intense grief reactions or role transitions (Miller et al. 2003).

The basic premise of cognitive-behavioral therapy is that depression is mediated by depressogenic patterns of thinking, which can be modified. Cognitive-behavioral therapy is considered useful for older depressed patients, but it requires vigilance in addressing hopelessness.

The available evidence upholds the effectiveness of psychological intervention with older adults, including the reduction of anxiety and management of insomnia (Barrowclough et al. 2001; Floyd and Scogin 1998; Knight and Satre 1999). Studies comparing younger with older psychotherapy patients found greater compliance in doing homework among younger individuals, but better attendance among older patients (Walker and Clarke 2001).

Problem-solving therapy in primary care has not yet proved itself superior to antidepressant medication. Further work is needed, because many older women may wish to receive treatment for depression at the primary level setting as a result of mobility problems (Williams et al. 2000).

Healthy Aging

Women tend to define healthy aging in terms of relationships. A group of women age 45 or older participating in a focus group proposed that a first step toward improving emotional well-being would be to work on building good relationships with partners, within the family, and with the community. Other strategies they suggested to boost resilience were to cultivate relational ties; value and nurture children, parents, and families; increase interpersonal and community connections; and promote equality for women (Kasle et al. 2002). The subjective experiences of menopause and aging arise through a multitude of factors that depend on individual personalities, coping skills, social support, and levels of neuroticism (Bosworth et al. 2003).

An integrated approach to healthy aging should focus on prevention and the indivisibility of physical and mental health, as proposed by the World Health Organization (1998). Collective efforts are needed to ensure that older women remain an active part of their community, participate in the planning and delivery of policies that affect their well-being, and transmit their knowledge and experience to younger generations.

Conclusion

Women live longer than before; they live longer than men. Their longevity challenges them to maintain adequate levels of health (healthy aging) while potentially exposed to several detrimental factors: multiple losses, increasing risks of physical disease, disabilities, discrimination, cognitive decline, depression, and dementia. The mental health practitioner, through social, pharmacological, and psychotherapeutic interventions and collaborative working relationships with other health care providers, can play a critical role in promoting health and ameliorating distress and psychiatric morbidity.

References

Abrams R, Spielman LA, Alexopoulos GS, et al: Personality disorder symptoms and functioning in elderly depressive patients. Am J Geriatr Psychiatry 6:24–30, 1998

Almeida OP, Fenner S: Bipolar disorder: similarities and differences between patients with illness onset before and after 65 years of age. Int Psychogeriatr 14:311–322, 2002

Alzheimer's Association: An overview of Alzheimer's disease: general statistics/demographics. Available at: http://www.alz.org/ResourceCenter/FactSheets/FSAlzheimerStats.pdf. Accessed May 16, 2003.

American Psychiatric Association: Diagnostic and Statistical Manual of Mental Disorders, 4th Edition, Text Revision. Washington, DC, American Psychiatric Association, 2000

Barrowclough C, King P, Colville J, et al: A randomized trial of the effectiveness of cognitive-behavioral therapy and supportive counseling for anxiety symptoms in older adults. J Consult Clin Psychol 69:756–762, 2001

Bergs D: "The Hidden Client"—women caring for husbands with COPD: their experience of quality of life. J Clin Nurs 11:613–621, 2002

Bonita R: Women, ageing and health. Available at the World Health Organization Ageing and Life Course Publications Web site: http://www.who.int/hpr/ageing/womenandageing.pdf. Accessed November 4, 2003.

Bosworth HB, Bastian LA, Rimer BK, et al: Coping styles and personality domains related to menopausal stress. Womens Health Issues 13:32–38, 2003

Bradley PJ: Family caregiver assessment: essential for effective home health care. J Gerontol Nurs 29:29–36, 2003

Cannuscio CC, Jones C, Kawachi I, et al: Reverberations of family illness: a longitudinal assessment of informal caregiving and mental health status in the Nurses' Health Study. Am J Public Health 92:1305–1311, 2002

Carrasco M: Trastornos de personalidad, in Psiquiatria Geriatrica. Edited by Agüera LF, Martín-Carrasco M, Cervilla JA. Barcelona, Masson, 2002

Charney DS, Reynolds CF III, Lewis L, et al: Depression and Bipolar Support Alliance consensus statement on the unmet needs in diagnosis and treatment of mood disorders in late life. Arch Gen Psychiatry 60:664–672, 2003

Denihan A, Kirby M, Bruce I, et al: Three-year prognosis of depression in the community-dwelling elderly. Br J Psychiatry 176:453–457, 2000

Depaola SJ, Griffin M, Young JR, et al: Death anxiety and attitudes toward the elderly among older adults: the role of gender and ethnicity. Death Stud 27:335–354, 2003

Devanand DP, Turret N, Moody BJ, et al: Personality disorders in elderly patients with dysthymic disorder. Am J Geriatr Psychiatry 8:188–195, 2000

Floyd M, Scogin F: Cognitive-behavior therapy for older adults: how does it work? Psychotherapy 35:459–463, 1998

Frank E, Frank N, Cornes C, et al: Interpersonal psychotherapy in the treatment of late life depression, in New Applications of Interpersonal Psychotherapy. Edited by Klerman G, Weissman M. Washington, DC, American Psychiatric Press, 1993, pp 167–198

Frasure-Smith N, Lespérance F, Talajic M: Depression and 18-month prognosis after myocardial infarction. Circulation 91:999–1005, 1995

Garner J: Psychodynamic work and older adults. Advances in Psychiatric Treatment 8:128–135, 2002

Geerlings M, Bouter L, Schoevers R, et al: Depression and risk of cognitive decline and Alzheimer's disease: results of two prospective community-based studies in the Netherlands. Br J Psychiatry 176:568–575, 2000

Gender and Aging Briefs, HelpAge International, 2000. Available at: http://www.helpage.org/images/pdfs/briefing%20papers/GenderPaper.PDF. Accessed June 2, 2002.

Henderson AS, Korten AE, Jacomb PA, et al: The course of depression in the elderly: a longitudinal community-based study in Australia. Psychol Med 27:119–129, 1997

Herbert J: Neurosteroids, brain damage, and mental illness. Exp Gerontol 33:713–727, 1998

Hooker K, Monahan DJ, Bowman SR, et al: Personality counts for a lot: predictors of mental and physical health of spouse caregivers in two disease groups. J Gerontol B Psychol Sci Soc Sci 53:73–85, 1998

Kasle S, Wilhelm MS, Reed KL: Optimal health and well-being for women: definitions and strategies derived from focus groups of women. Womens Health Issues 12:178–190, 2002

Kim JS: Daughters-in-law in Korean caregiving families. J Adv Nurs 36:399–408, 2001

Klausner EJ, Alexopoulos GS: The future of psychosocial treatments for elderly patients. Psychiatr Serv 50:1198–1204, 1999

Knight B, Satre DD: Cognitive behavioral psychotherapy with older adults. Clinical Psychology: Science and Practice 62:188–203, 1999

Laidlaw TM, Coverdale JH, Falloon IR, et al: Caregivers' stresses when living together or apart from patients with chronic schizophrenia. Community Ment Health J 38:303–310, 2002

Levkoff SE, Evans DA, Liptzin B, et al: Delirium: the occurrence and persistence of symptoms among elderly hospitalized patients. Arch Intern Med 152:334–340, 1992

Li C, Wilawan K, Samsioe G, et al: Health profile of middle-aged women: the Women's Health in the Lund Area (WHILA) study. Hum Reprod 17:1379–1385, 2002

Lokkegaard E, Pedersen AT, Laursen P, et al: The influence of hormone replacement therapy on the aging-related change in cognitive performance: analysis based on a Danish cohort study. Maturitas 42:209–218, 2002

MacDonald W, Nemeroff CF: Practical guidelines for diagnosing and treating bipolar disorder in the elderly. Medscape Psychiatry and Mental Health eJournal 3(2), 1998. Available at http://www.medscape.com/viewarticle/430757. Accessed June 2, 2002.

Marcuccio E, Loving N, Bennett SK, et al: A survey of attitudes and experiences of women with heart disease. Womens Health Issues 13:23–31, 2003

Martire LM, Stephens MA, Townsend AL: Centrality of women's multiple roles: beneficial and detrimental consequences for psychological well-being. Psychology and Aging 15:148–156, 2000

Mayeaux R: Predicting who will develop Alzheimer's disease, in Epidemiology of Alzheimer's Disease: From Gene to Prevention. Edited by Mayeaux R, Christen Y. New York, Springer-Verlag, 1999, pp 19–31

McLay RN, Maki PM, Lyketsos CG: Nulliparity and late menopause are associated with decreased cognitive decline. J Neuropsychiatry Clin Neurosci 15:161–167, 2003

Meagher D: Delirium: the role of psychiatry. Adv Psychiatr Treat 7:433–434, 2001

Miller MD, Cornes C, Frank E, et al: Interpersonal psychotherapy for late-life depression: past, present, and future. J Psychother Pract Res 10:231–238, 2001

Miller MD, Frank E, Cornes C, et al: The value of maintenance interpersonal psychotherapy (IPT) in older adults with different IPT foci. Am J Geriatr Psychiatry 11:97–102, 2003

Nestadt G, Bienvenu OJ, Cai G, et al: Incidence of obsessive-compulsive disorder in adults. J Nerv Ment Dis 186:401–406, 1998

Paoletti I: A half life: women caregivers of older disabled relatives. J Women Aging 11:53–67, 1999

Petrovic M, Vandierendonck A, Mariman A, et al: Personality traits and socio-epidemiological status of hospitalised elderly benzodiazepine users. Int J Geriatr Psychiatry 17:733–738, 2002

Pinquart M, Sorensen S: Differences between caregivers and noncaregivers in psychological health and physical health: a meta-analysis. Psychol Aging 18:250–267, 2003

Rapp SR, Espeland MA, Shumaker SA, et al: Effect of estrogen plus progestin on global cognitive function in postmenopausal women: the Women's Health Initiative Memory Study: a randomized controlled trial. WHIMS Investigators. JAMA 289:2663–2672, 2003

Schoevers RA, Geerlings MI, Beekman AT, et al: Association of depression and gender with mortality in old age: results from the Amsterdam Study of the Elderly (AMSTEL). Br J Psychiatry 177:336–342, 2000

Sherif T, Jehani T, Saadani M, et al: Adult oncology and chronically ill patients: comparison of depression, anxiety and caregivers' quality of life. East Mediterr Health J 7:502–509, 2001

Sherwin BB: Sex hormones and psychological functioning in postmenopausal women. Exp Gerontol 29:423–430, 1994

Shulman KI, Rochon P, Sykora K, et al: Changing prescription patterns for lithium and valproic acid in old age: shifting practice without evidence. BMJ 326:960–961, 2003

Shumaker SA, Legault C, Rapp SR, et al: Estrogen plus progestin and the incidence of dementia and mild cognitive impairment in postmenopausal women: the Women's Health Initiative Memory Study: a randomized controlled trial. JAMA 289:2651–2662, 2003

Stein MB, Barrett-Connor E: Quality of life in older adults receiving medications for anxiety, depression, or insomnia: findings from a community-based study. Am J Geriatr Psychiatry 10:568–574, 2002

Swar S: Statement by Nepal at the Second World Assembly on Ageing, Madrid. Available at: http://www.un.org/ageing/coverage/nepalE.htm. Accessed May 16, 2003.

Veltman A, Cameron J, Stewart DE: The experience of providing care to relatives with chronic mental illness. J Nerv Ment Dis 190:108–114, 2002

Walker DA, Clarke M: Cognitive behavioral psychotherapy: a comparison between younger and older adults in two inner city mental health teams. Aging Ment Health 5:197–199, 2001

Wallace Williams S, Dilworth-Anderson P, Goodwin PY: Caregiver role strain: the contribution of multiple roles and available resources in African-American women. Aging Ment Health 7:103–112, 2003

Williams JW, Barrett J, Oxman T, et al: Treatment of dysthymia and minor depression in primary care: a randomized controlled trial in older adults. JAMA 284:1519–1526, 2000

World Health Organization: The role of physical activity in healthy ageing. WHO/HPR/AHE/98.1, 1998, pp. 5–6. Available at: http://www.who.int/hpr/ageing/roleofphysactiv.pdf. Accessed November 5, 2004.

World Health Organization: Towards policy for health and ageing. Available at: http://www.who.int/hpr/ageing/ageing.pdf. Accessed June 2, 2002a.

World Health Organization: Women, ageing and health (Fact sheet 252). Geneva, World Health Organization, 2002b

Xavier FM, Ferraza MP, Argimon I, et al: The DSM-IV "minor depression" disorder in the oldest-old: prevalence rate, sleep patterns, memory function and quality of life in elderly people of Italian descent in Southern Brazil. Int J Geriatr Psychiatry 17:107–116, 2002

Index

*Page numbers printed in **boldface** type refer to tables or figures.*